# The Physician Within

# The Physician Within

## A Step-by-Step Guide to Living Well with Chronic Illness

### Catherine Feste

*Nov 1, 1996*

*To Sara*

♡

*Cathy Feste*

An Owl Book

Henry Holt and Company
New York

Henry Holt and Company, Inc.
*Publishers since 1866*
115 West 18th Street
New York, New York 10011

Henry Holt® is a registered trademark
of Henry Holt and Company, Inc.

Published in Canada by Fitzhenry & Whiteside Ltd.,
195 Allstate Parkway, Markham, Ontario L3R 4T8.

Library of Congress Cataloging-in-Publication Data
Feste, Catherine.
The physician within: a step-by-step guide to living well
with chronic illness / Catherine Feste.—1st Owl book ed.
p.   cm.
Originally published: Minneapolis, Chronimed Pub., 1993.
"An Owl book."
Includes index.
1. Chronic diseases—Psychological aspects.
2. Chronically ill—Health and hygiene.   3. Sick—Psychology.
4. Medicine, Psychosomatic.   I. Title.
RC108.F47   1995                                95-15194
616.001'9—dc20                                      CIP

ISBN 0-8050-3951-1

Henry Holt books are available for special promotions
and premiums. For details contact: Director, Special Markets.

First published in 1993 by Chronimed Publishing.

First Owl Book Edition—1995

Printed in the United States of America
All first editions are printed on acid-free paper.∞

1   3   5   7   9   10   8   6   4   2

## Dedication

For her wisdom, love
and never-ending support,
this book is lovingly
dedicated
to my
mother

# ACKNOWLEDGMENTS

Bob Anderson is a mentor, teacher, kindred spirit, and friend. His vision of empowerment and his depth of human understanding reinforced my own. My gratitude is expressed for his critical review of the empowerment chapter, his reading of the entire manuscript, and the years of professional enrichment and support.

Kathy Plumb is the personification of empowerment. Integrating great physical challenges into her life, she has inspired and taught all of us that life is a celebration. She reviewed the empowerment chapter, but before that, her life gave validity to the whole concept.

Since the first edition of this book was published, I had the exciting experience of having a fellowship at the International Diabetes Institute in Melbourne, Australia. I am indebted to the wonderful staff with whom I worked and learned, especially Paul Zimmet, Matt Cohen, Christine Crosbie, and Cathie Roby.

Thank you to John Valusek, Ph.D., founder of People Are Not For Hitting, for his critical review of the empowerment chapter. I am especially grateful for John's mission, which teaches that empowerment comes from love, not violence.

Throughout most of my professional life, my collegial base has been the members of the American Association of Diabetes Educators. Their commitment to educational excellence and service to others has guided me.

Affiliates of the ADA have provided me a venue for teaching. My thanks to the many people I have met who shared their successful coping techniques and their tireless commitment to living and loving each day of their lives.

My deep gratitude goes to Alice Ring, MD, MPH, and her colleagues at the Centers for Disease Control for their support and for their leadership in prevention.

Dee Ready taught me why stories are important: "Stories clothe theory in humanity."

Pat Lassonde did the superb editorial job with this book. Beyond that, Pat has been a mentor, guide, and inspiration as she has shared with me how she has successfully adapted rheumatoid arthritis into her life.

# TABLE OF CONTENTS

## FOREWORD

I have just finished reading *The Physician Within*. I feel better now about what I can do to generate well-being within myself, even though I don't have diabetes or any other chronic disease.

How could this happen to a gruff physician trained in the mechanistic school of medicine? After all, doesn't disease derive from aberrations which, when corrected, result in the resumption of health? Who is better able to restore health than physicians? They sift through signs and symptoms to reach a diagnosis and, on the basis of understanding the pathophysiology, institute treatment that, in and of itself, should correct the underlying disorder. In this stilted view, the patient is merely the vehicle of disease and a passive recipient of treatment. All that is required of the patient is to comply with the treatment, and cure or control of disease is effected.

How simplistic and naive! Many of us physicians, however, have been guilty of reducing management of disease to these very terms. With the passage of time and with even the smallest chink open to faint rays of wisdom, we gradually come to appreciate that our role in disease management is that of a partner with patients wherein their contribution to their own well-being usually exceeds that of the physician. Good health and feeling well, just as ill health and not feeling well, do not inevitably coexist.

*The Physician Within* elucidates in a richly anecdotal and warmly robust fashion the power innate in all of us to deal effectively with chronic disease. Since physicians often do not have the training nor the time to awaken and nurture within the patient the spirit, confidence, self-reliance, optimism, and self-improvement necessary for his or her successful adaptation to chronic disease, *The Physician Within* provides an essential component to a comprehensive treatment program.

*F. John Service, M.D., Ph.D.*
*Division of Endocrinology and Metabolism*
*Mayo Clinic, Rochester, Minnesota*

The seed for this book was planted in 1957, when I was diagnosed as having diabetes. That began my personal excursion into well-being. My professional interest in well-being began in the early 1970s, when I was the education director for the Minnesota affiliate of the American Diabetes Association. In that position I observed a great disparity among people with diabetes. Some became angry and bitter and sort of dropped out of life. Others took their diabetes in stride and continued to enjoy a fulfilling and enjoyable life. The difference did not seem to be related to anything physical. Some with the greatest physical problems had the biggest smiles on their faces.

My study began. My research question was: "Why do people do well?" I studied healthy people everywhere. They were "healthy people" who had diabetes, cancer, arthritis, or some other great life challenges such as the loss of a limb, spouse, or child. The common denominator was that they were all survivors. They chose to keep going instead of giving up. They chose to gracefully incorporate their challenge into their lives, neither making battle with it nor ignoring it. They didn't fit the popular image of "diabetics," "arthritics," "epileptics," or "cripples." They continued to be active, happy individuals who happen to have a health challenge.

The more I studied these people the more exciting this work became. I observed some unmistakable common threads in the fabric of their lives. The threads are these three concepts: COPE, SUPPORT, and HOPE. (The psycho/social/spiritual dimension.) By weaving those threads together, I developed a lecture-discussion series that became the basis for this book.

This book is about the unique and powerful well-being that people attain when they use their inner resources to cope successfully with a challenge. I have not described every challenge, but I have described the process I believe leads to a fulfilling sense of well-being no matter what the individual challenge may be. No book, person, or organization can tell you how to live well. Each individual must discover how to do that for himself or herself. THIS BOOK PROVIDES A STRUCTURE TO SUPPORT YOUR SELF-DISCOVERY.

When your AWARENESS leads to responsible CHOICES, then you are empowered. In this revised edition of *The Physician Within,* we have added a chapter on empowerment and updated the other chapters to reflect and encourage empowerment. Empowerment springs from the unique experience of the individual, which connects us to the universal experience of being human. With that in mind, in this new edition, I have shared more of my personal stories. This was done to encourage you to connect with your own. Stories told from the heart go directly to another's heart.

Our stories may be quite different in circumstance and content—but the core messages unite us. One person's discovery of hope is made in a hospice while another's is in a ghetto. Different people, having diverse experiences, discovering the same hope. In this way, we make connections with one another and with all humanity.

This book has at least three possible uses.

1. You may choose to read it and reflect on it alone.

2. You may wish to use it as a guide for discussions with your various advisors and supporters.

3. You may want to use any portion but especially the reflection and discussion questions at the end of each chapter as the basis for group discussions. No matter how you use it, remember that the whole purpose is to enhance your well-being.

I know of no more encouraging fact than the unquestionable ability of man to elevate his life by a conscious endeavor.

—Henry David Thoreau

Wishing you lifelong well-being,

Catherine Feste

# The Physician Within

# A
# *Lifetime of*
# *Well-Being*

*Health and intellect are the two blessings of life.*
Menander 342-292 B.C.

Menander's observation, made hundreds of years before Christ, may be the first of many assertions that health is the greatest blessing. Throughout history, when people have suffered great material loss, a frequent comment has been: "Well, we have our health. That's what's important."

What does it mean, then, when health is threatened by a disease or a deviation from what is generally regarded as healthy? (Such deviations can include weight loss or gain, pain, or other symptoms that occur without the diagnosis of a disease.) Does the presence of a health problem mean that we have been robbed of one of life's greatest blessings?

Absolutely not. There are millions of wonderfully *healthy* people who happen to have arthritis, diabetes, high blood pressure, heart problems, lupus, multiple sclerosis. The list can go on and on. But despite their disease, these people enjoy *well-being*. Menander was getting at well-being when he included intellect with health. But he separated the two. Well-being implies a more comprehensive view of health than simply the physical. Well-being includes health of the mind, emotions, and spirit.

In order to regain well-being after the onset of a health problem, and then to maintain that well-being to the end of one's life, each of us can explore questions like these:

**What does well-being mean? How well am I? How can I either regain or reinforce my well-being? Where can I get support for my well-being?**

Each of us defines well-being differently, but some elements of well-being appear in a variety of definitions:

> Having a purpose in life
> Feeling in control of life
> Sharing life's ups and downs with friends
> Feeling capable of handling life's ups and downs
> Having fun
> Feeling good about who I am
> Helping others
> Believing that I make a contribution to life
> Feeling loved and lovable
> Experiencing peace and joy

Believing that life is worthwhile
Having hope

Many life events can threaten our sense of well-being. Losing a job or experiencing the loss of a personal relationship can threaten just about all of the elements listed above. Getting a new job or seeking a new relationship may lessen these threats to well being, but disease cannot be divorced or resigned from. It must be made part of your life. **The vital question is whether you succeed in making it part of an overall healthy life or whether it overcomes your pursuit of well-being.** The objective of this book is to encourage you to discover how to integrate your chronic disease into your life without sacrificing the quality of your life. This book looks at living with a chronic disease while actively pursuing a fulfilling life.

As I explored well-being I found that it is an approach to life. Along with many other people with health challenges, I discovered that the highest level of well-being is not something you achieve *in spite* of suffering; it is something you attain *because* of suffering.

Out of suffering have emerged the strongest souls;
the most massive characters are seared with scars.

E.H. Chapin

Once you have explored well-being and how to achieve it, you will have the choice of whether or not it becomes your overall approach to life. Following are two case studies. Both girls have similar values and ambitions: to enjoy life as a teenager! And both girls have diabetes. As you read these case studies, try to identify the elements that make one girl's approach that of well-being and the other's that of a helpless victim of circumstances.

## Case study #1

Sandy is 17 years old. She has had diabetes since she was 14. She has not told many of her friends she has diabetes. She does not want to be considered different from them. She understands what diabetes requires of her, but she resents what she calls its "demands." So sometimes she does not bring a snack with her when she is to be gone in the afternoon.

One day Sandy and a friend planned to go boating at the friend's lake cabin. Sandy packed suntan lotion, towel, bathing suit, and straw hat, but, self-conscious about her special needs, she did not pack food either for her afternoon snack or for a possible insulin reaction.

Sandy and her friend arrived at the lake and immediately went out in the boat. They listened to the radio, chatted, and sunbathed. By 3 p.m. Sandy began to feel a bit shaky. She looked in her friend's cooler and found only sugar-free soda pop. She was beginning to have an insulin reaction, and she had nothing with sugar in it so she could boost her falling blood sugar.

Sandy's friend had to quickly drive the boat back to their cabin where, fortunately, they had some sugar left from the previous summer. But what if there had been nothing there?

Sandy's response to the situation was, "That darned diabetes! It's always getting in my way. I can't have 'normal' fun like my friends do. I hate having diabetes."

## Case study #2

Lucy is 15 years old and has had diabetes since she was 10. She tells her friends about diabetes, but she doesn't make a big deal out of it. She explains what she has to do and why, then goes about her life.

One morning Lucy and a friend decided to go shopping. Realizing there would be plenty of food available at the mall, Lucy reasoned: "If I need a snack or something for low blood sugar, I can always buy something, but I should have some food with me 'just in case.' " So Lucy packed a small can of juice and a bag of graham crackers.

Lucy and her friend took the city bus to the shopping center, where they shopped and walked a lot. At 11 a.m. they took the bus over to another shopping center to have lunch and shop a bit more before returning home. But soon after boarding, Lucy began to feel lightheaded and sweaty. She was beginning to have an insulin reaction. Confidently, she reached into her bag for the juice. She drank it and ate a graham cracker. By the time they reached the shopping center, Lucy felt fine again, and they both forgot about the brief incident of low blood sugar. They remember that day as a lot of fun.

Now, comparing the two incidents, what suggestions would you make to change the unhealthy situation to a healthy one? Think of an incident relating to your own health challenge. See yourself in a social, family, or work situation. Discuss why it is difficult to handle certain situations with a positive attitude and healthy behavior. Now, discuss how that situation can be handled with a spirit of well-being.

Living well with a challenge is the thrust of this entire book. Life brings many challenges: growing up, getting a job, changing jobs, losing a job, getting married, losing your spouse, moving to a different part of the country, rearing children, caring for aging parents . . . and getting a disease, which is the challenge on which this book will focus. Since challenges simply cannot be avoided, we must learn how to live well with them.

Novelist and poet Robert Louis Stevenson had tuberculosis all his life. Despite it, he lived adventurously and traveled widely. Of this challenge he said, "Life is not a matter of holding good cards. It's playing a poor hand well." That spirit of determination can guide each of us to live well with any challenge life brings.

The medical aspect of living well with a disease can come from the advice of a knowledgeable, skilled, and caring medical team. A good team teaches clients the healthy behaviors to follow in order to control the disease or the effects of it. For you to be motivated to follow the advice of your medical team, you need to approach life with the attitude that you *can* and *will* live a life of well-being. One of the most important aspects of this attitude is the belief that life is worthwhile. Medical advisors can tell you *how* to live; you must supply the important *why*.

The essence of living well with your disease is your answer to these questions: Why do you want to live well? What makes your life worthwhile? The answer to your *why* will motivate you to follow the *how*.

Philosopher Friedrich Nietzsche ventured even further when he said, "He who has a why to live can bear almost any how."

## Approach all challenges well

When people get a disease, the approach they take to the disease usually reflects their basic approach to life. Janet and Dorothy are interesting examples of this point.

Janet is a 37-year-old secretary. She has worked at a large insurance company for 15 years. One day she was told by her boss that she was being considered for a promotion. She declined the promotion, saying she was really too old to get into something new, to learn all that would be required. She didn't think she could handle it.

There is nothing medically wrong with Janet, but she does complain of being tired most of the time, so she turns down many invitations from friends. Not only does she lack energy, she also lacks enthusiasm for hobbies, projects, her work, even her family. Janet is not ill. But is she well?

Dorothy is a 50-year-old widow with three teenaged children. She works outside the home to support her family. She would prefer to stay home, but she must work to help support her family, so she has chosen to make the best of it. She approaches her work with enthusiasm instead of resignation. She is looking into further schooling for herself, realizing that once her children leave home she will need to have meaningful, enjoyable, fulfilling activity in her life.

Within six months of one another, Janet and Dorothy both are told they have cancer. How do you think each responded to it? Which one thought of it as "the end of the world"? Which one looked at it as a "challenge I can handle"? Which one used it as an excuse to not do things? Which one sought the best medical and educational advice so as to "get the best of it so it won't get the best of me"?

Two years later, Janet has transferred all her negative feelings about life to her cancer. It used to be her "rotten job" that made her tired and irritable. Now it's her "lousy cancer." Even though her chemotherapy causes her to feel ill only occasionally, Janet complains constantly that she doesn't feel well, doesn't have any energy, can't work, can't see friends, etc. Her lack of energy is blown out of proportion in terms of what is caused by cancer or its treatment. Janet is undeniably ill, but so is her whole approach to life.

Dorothy is a sharp contrast to Janet. She gets the same chemotherapy as Janet, and it does sap her energy for a while. Instead of complaining as Janet does, Dorothy adjusts her lifestyle to accommodate her low energy days. She fills those days with activities she can handle and does not complain about how she feels. On the days she feels well she functions absolutely normally. She shares her simple philosophy: "I savor the good days and make the most of each moment when I feel well. I never look back at the days of illness. I only look forward to the activities I enjoy: seeing my friends, being with my family, doing my work, and giving to my community."

Dorothy and Janet have the same doctor. He feels very optimistic about Dorothy's chances of doing well but is concerned about Janet's future. Doctors have understood for many years that attitude plays an important role in healing. Dorothy's upbeat, forward-thinking, positive attitude will serve her well.

For Janet and Dorothy, well-being has nothing to do with a physical state of being. Long before each got cancer, each demonstrated her basic approach to life.

Dorothy's approach illustrates an observation many people have made over the years. Individuals who do well with any disease tend to believe that life is too worthwhile to give up just because they have a disease. When disease or adversity strikes these people, they simply do not allow it to interrupt their life. Their desire to continue living a satisfying life inspires them to figure out how to work their disease into their life.

It is natural to focus on your disease when you are first diagnosed and also whenever it becomes the center of your attention. This can occur because your health has worsened or changed, you've applied for a job, you've heard or read a story about someone who has the same disease, or whatever. But when disease becomes the focus of your life rather than something to be integrated into a healthy, whole life, you must remind yourself of what you mean by a healthy whole life. To help you regain your perspective, fill out the following Life Satisfaction Survey. Doing this will not only help you see that your life is much more than your disease, it will also help you find problem areas that can be causing you stress.

## Life Satisfaction Survey

Evaluate your satisfaction with life by responding to the following with an X under SA (Strongly agree), A (Agree), D (Disagree), SD (Strongly disagree).

| Physical | SA | A | D | SD |
|---|---|---|---|---|
| I think of myself as generally healthy. | | | | |
| My weight is where I want it to be. | | | | |
| My exercise program is satisfactory to me. | | | | |
| My eating habits are nutritionally sound. | | | | |
| **Mental** | | | | |
| I manage stress well. | | | | |
| I am seldom depressed. | | | | |
| I feel sufficiently stimulated mentally. | | | | |
| **Spiritual** | | | | |
| I am at peace with myself and the world around me. | | | | |
| I can experience joy. | | | | |
| I can experience love. | | | | |
| I feel hopeful about the future. | | | | |
| **Family** | | | | |
| **(If you have no family, apply this to friends.)** | | | | |
| I have close, loving family relationships. | | | | |
| My family supports me. | | | | |
| I support the members of my family. | | | | |
| **Social** | | | | |
| I have friends in whom I can confide. | | | | |
| My friends care about me. | | | | |
| I give support to my friends. | | | | |
| My friends support me. | | | | |

| Work-related | SA | A | D | SD |
|---|---|---|---|---|
| I am in the right job. | | | | |
| I feel capable in my work. | | | | |
| I feel valued for what I do. | | | | |
| I look forward to going to work. | | | | |
| **Financial** | | | | |
| I have enough money for what I need. | | | | |
| I have no serious financial worries. | | | | |
| I have planned for retirement. | | | | |
| **Personal** | | | | |
| I take time for myself. | | | | |
| I engage in enjoyable leisure activities. | | | | |
| Overall, I am satisfied with my life. | | | | |

Keeping in mind that it is both normal and healthy to experience some dissatisfaction, please look at the areas with which you have the greatest dissatisfaction. These are the areas that will provide you with goals to work on to increase the level of satisfaction in your life. At times, however, you can feel great dissatisfaction with much of your life. If your life is so unsatisfactory that the survey has left you feeling overwhelmed or hopeless, then please seek help from a counselor who can assist you in establishing helpful goals. Then come back to this book for reinforcement as you continue your ongoing journey toward well-being.

Select two or three areas you want to start with in the goal-setting process.

1. Choose a goal that is important to you. You will be more motivated to work on a goal *you* have chosen rather than one someone else has chosen for you. To choose health-related goals, have an open, candid discussion with your medical team. Any health-related goal is a team effort. Your team can give you important information about your disease, and you can share important information about your life. Good outcomes can only be achieved when disease and life are integrated. Your medical advisors are experts in the one, and you are the expert in the other. The goals they have for you and the goals you set for yourself ought to aim at the same outcome: maximizing the quality of your life.

2. Goals should be *specific* and *measurable*. Instead of saying, "I want to lose weight," decide how much you want to lose. Ten pounds, for instance, is a measurable and specific amount, so you will know when you have achieved your goal.

3. Goals must be *time-dated*. "I am going to lose ten pounds" is a goal you could have for 20 years or more! "I will lose one pound a week for ten weeks" is an example of a specific, time-dated goal.

4. Goals should be *evaluated* regularly. If you did not lose that pound this week it may have been unrealistic for some reason, or there may be an obstacle that you must deal with before you can proceed to attain your goal. Let others help in the evaluation. Any health-related goal should be discussed with and followed up by your medical team. Goals that involve friends or family members may benefit from their evaluation. As you look at any of your goals, think

about experts who can assist you in evaluating your goal. But ultimately it will be your gut level intuition that will probably guide you the best in evaluating.

5. Reward your behavior instead of results. A positive result will be its own wonderful reward when it happens. But to keep you going, reward the behaviors that will take you to that end result. One of the benefits of rewarding healthy behaviors occurs when they become part of your life. When you focus only on results, you drop the healthy behaviors as soon as the result has been attained and return to old, negative behavior. Then eventually the result is lost as well. This is one explanation for the "yo-yo" phenomenon in weight loss. In concentrating only on weight loss and not on behavior change, people lose weight only to quickly put it back on.

The more you understand about your goals and your*self,* the more likely you are to succeed. Reflect on the following questions:

- What am I willing to change to achieve this goal?
- Have I failed to achieve this goal before? Why?
- What will I do differently this time to enhance my success?
- Am I really committed to working on this goal until it is achieved?

In another chapter we will explore problem solving. Working on goals is a good way to uncover problems. A walk through the neighborhood is a great exercise goal, until it rains. Besides problem solving you will find the upcoming chapters contain practical, helpful information to assist you in achieving your overall goal of well-being.

You will be invited to explore your **self-image** to see if it is life-enhancing. If your exploration indicates a self-image that needs some improvement, you will find practical suggestions to help you.

**Motivation** is another element in a healthy life. In exploring your motivation, you will examine all the forces around and within you that influence decisions you make. If you discover you are not satisfied with those forces, you can explore ways to control them and thus take a more direct role in making your own choices.

Because life is constantly changing, you will need the tool of **adaptability** to help you discover how you can adjust to change without sacrificing the quality of your life.

Stress is part of life, but with **stress management** tools you can make choices that will prevent stress from seriously interrupting your pursuit of a fulfilling life. In the stress management chapter you will also be asked to explore a technique designed to prevent stress from taking control of you.

**Problem solving** is explored as a practical step-by-step process, useful for overcoming problems presented by a chronic disease. The process is equally useful as an approach to any problem, and so it reinforces the philosophy you will find in each chapter. This is about LIFE. Our challenges vary, but the skills and tools we use are part of a healthy life.

And healthy lives are supported. In the **support** chapter you will explore what support means to you, how you like to get it, and what you need to do to get it.

The Physician Within is **hope**, the spiritual component of a healthy life. You're invited to explore your resources and gain insight into how you can activate this aspect of your life.

The **empowerment** chapter asks you to explore how you make your choices: the *freedom* you have to choose how you will live your life and the *responsibility* you have for the choices you make.

As you explore your choices you may see a **plan of action** evolve. It is both freeing and frustrating to realize that the plan we make for our lives is truly a "living document." It must change as we adapt to what life brings.

Once you understand that, you can accept life as truly a process— the proverbial "journey" rather than a destination. As challenges arise you can reconnect with your resources: a healthy self-image, the ability to take control of your own motivation, the capacity to adapt to life's changes, stress management and problem solving techniques, the support around you, and the support within you. By employing all of these resources in your behalf you will be empowered to experience and enjoy a **lifetime of well-being.**

The process used to take you on your journey can be described by these four words: explore, reflect, apply, evaluate. As you read this book and live your life, be aware of this process.

EXPLORE the information presented in this book and at the same time explore your life. Continue your exploration by seeking other books or classes or people with whom you can discuss these and similar ideas.

REFLECT on all that you are learning about yourself. Reflection takes time, space, and solitude. Set aside some time. Select a space conducive to this activity—a favorite place—whether that's the rocking chair on the front proch, a favorite stuffed chair in your living room, or the country road where you take your daily walk. Solitude may require that you get up before the rest of the family or that you travel to a spot where you can be undisturbed. So not skip over the reflection step by moving directly to application from exploration. Reflection leads to insight. It's important to process what you're learning. Run it through the filter of your life experiences, needs, and goals. Then, apply the insights gained through this process.

APPLY the information you have gathered to yourself. Trust your intuition to tell you what is most likely to be helpful to you. At the same time, don't be afraid to try something new. A technique that may have struck you as unlikely to be of any help a few years ago may today hold promise of great benefit. (The technique of journaling became an exciting adventure for a nurse who initially viewed it as a classroom writing assignment.)

Finally, EVALUATE. Was this new skill helpful to you? If not, explore some more. Find another insight into your challenge and a technique for addressing it. Apply that. And evaluate. Never stop exploring, reflecting, applying, and evaluating.

## Summary

• Well-being is an approach to life that allows you to live well with all the challenges life presents.

• The medical aspect of living well comes from being a part of a knowledgeable, skilled, and caring medical team.

• Surveying your life to measure how satisfied you are with its various dimensions will help you discover what you mean by a healthy, whole life and to set goals in areas that need attention.

• How you approach living with a disease usually reflects your basic approach to life. A person who is committed to making the most out of life will be inspired to figure out how to continue to live well with disease. Skills that must be developed and continually sharpened in order to live well with a disease include: positive self-image, motivation, adaptability, stress management, problem solving, and getting support from others.

• The spiritual component of a healthy life is your "Physician Within." However you define it in your life, it is the force that undergirds and sustains you in the face of a challenge.

• A Plan of Action is a vital tool for using skills to achieve a personal file of well-being.

## Reflection Questions

1. Identify elements that describe your sense of well-being. (Refer to the bottom of page 2.)

2. Describe your current greatest threat to your well-being or to your purpose in life. (Be specific in identifying which elements of your well-being you feel are "under fire.")
3. Identify the area(s) in the Life Satisfaction survey you want to start with in the goal-setting process.

Write your goals here:

Are these important to you?
Are these specific and measurable?
Are these time dated?
How will you evaluate your goals?
How will you reward yourself?

As you read this book, keep focusing on both

1. Your definition of well-being, and

2. The threat you feel to your well-being.

As you read each chapter, look for ways to overcome the threat and identify ways to reinforce your sense of well-being.

# CHAPTER 2

# Self-Image: Taking Charge of Who You Are

Self-image is a powerful force in our lives. Who you *think* you are determines what you do and how you feel about yourself. How you *feel* about yourself has a great influence on how people react to you. Negative self-image plays a major role in child abuse, spouse abuse, divorce, crimes, in virtually all the failures of humanity. On the other hand, positive self-image plays a large role in whether you succeed in life, and it also enables you to nurture those around you.

One type of success that depends greatly on self-image is the ability to continue to believe in your self-worth following the onset of a disease or disability. Self-image is your armor, your defense against careless remarks, ("Oh, how long have you been crippled?"); ugly words and labels (deaf and dumb, spastic, arthritic, and diabetic); and the many negative messages that assault you daily. Self-image is also the powerful, positive vision that helps you not only to rise above the negative images, but more important, to gain self-confidence and to be at peace with who you are.

This chapter focuses on understanding the source and function of self-image and suggests techniques that can help you enhance your self-image and gain greater control over it. This will be a practical, down-to-earth approach to a highly complex issue. It starts with the premise that everyone's self-image can stand a boost.

For this approach to work, you must already have a fairly healthy self-esteem or sense of self-worth. If you have difficulty using the techniques in this chapter, you may need some professional help to "get the ball rolling." Evaluate yourself as you read and give the suggestions an honest try. If they don't help and your negative self-image won't budge, then you need more than this book can give you. You not only need more, you deserve more. Don't give up on yourself. Go to resources such as your physician, a family counselor, clergyperson, or a similar trusted advisor who can guide you toward getting the help you need to develop your positive and healthy self-image. Then come back to this chapter for reinforcement.

## What is your self-image today?

What words would you use to describe yourself? Put a check mark by the words in the following list that you feel describe you:

| | |
|---|---|
| thoughtful | indestructible |
| self-confident | friendly |
| lazy | stupid |
| courageous | weak |
| generous | dishonest |
| assertive | honest |
| healthy | sickly |
| shy | trustworthy |
| fearful | a loser |
| successful | a winner |
| passive | unsure |
| loving | tough |
| attractive | caring |
| second best | ill |
| fortunate | tenacious |
| impulsive | out of control |

Now, on a separate sheet of paper list your strengths and weaknesses as you see them. Remember that everyone has strengths. Be as generous with your self-appraisal as you would be in appraising a friend.

Did you find it easier to list your weaknesses than your strengths? If you did, you are in the majority. Most people do. Be sure that you have not short-changed yourself. You do have strengths. Make another list of the strengths that your greatest supporters (friends, mother, boss, neighbor, etc.) would say you have. These lists will give you some insight into your self-image.

This insight may or may not be an accurate description of who you really are. It is significant, though, because it is what you *think* you are. And what you think you are affects what you do.

People behave in a manner consistent with their self-image. For example, most smokers view themselves as smokers. In successful smoking cessation treatment using hypnosis, people are given the hypnotic suggestion that they are nonsmokers. This has helped people to quit smoking. Their self-image has changed: Why would a nonsmoker even buy cigarettes?

Overweight people find themselves losing weight when they cease to view themselves as fat and instead think of themselves as slender—and eat accordingly. Self-image serves very much like a blueprint for behavior. That's why it is so important to have as positive a self-image as you possibly can.

## Yesterday created today's self-image

One of the earliest and most significant influences on self-image is the message you got about yourself from your parents. Parents are like mirrors to which their children look to learn about themselves. By gaining parental approval, children gain self-approval. The message for a child is, "If my parents like me, then I must be a worthwhile person."

This concept is not universally understood. Some parents believe that if they give their children compliments and other positive feedback, their children will become egotistical and "spoiled." Thus, nurturing comments like "I love you," "I like you," or "You're a thoughtful girl," are withheld. This is unfortunate because these kinds of comments develop a healthy personality and a positive self-image. Even sadder than withholding positive comments is the giving of negative comments like "You dummy,"

"You're so clumsy," "You lazy slob," or "Hey, stupid!" These messages of early childhood—both positive and negative— become the basis for a person's self-image. The actions of our parents also have a great influence on our self-image.

Our parents' behavior sends strong messages for our lives. If they tolerate cruelty, we abuse others. If they convey affection, we feel loved. If they demonstrate sloppiness, we never learn to take care of ourselves. If they limit our destructiveness, we learn self-control. If they act courageously, we feel strong. If they are deceitful, we learn not to trust others. If they are active, we become participants. If they are hypochondriacs, we become sickly ourselves. If they make excuses for mistakes, we don't learn to take responsibility for our actions. We *think* we are like our parents, and therefore, we *learn* to live in the good or bad ways they demonstrate. I like the way Haim Ginott expresses this concept:

> Children are like wet cement. Whatever falls
> on them makes an impression.

A person's self-image can be created not only by parents, but also by such authority figures as teachers, health professionals, and clergy, and by relatives such as aunts, uncles, and grandparents. Richly blessed is the adult who lived among nurturing adults while growing up. The healthy person leaves this loving environment of adult approval feeling so self-confident that he or she can take on the task of self-nurturing and approval giving. The positive self-image serves a function similar to that of a coach. When your parents are no longer doing the coaching and encouraging, you can look to your own internal coach for approval and advice. The person with a positive self-image finds a coach who *forgives* shortcomings (no one is perfect); *encourages* one's finest efforts (reach for excellence, falling short is better than not trying); and *loves* unconditionally (no matter what, you are a worthwhile person).

Children's minds are like tape recorders. They absorb what they see and hear and tend to believe indiscriminately all the messages to which they are exposed. Those tapes stay with you forever unless you challenge them and change them. A confident and capable executive confessed that he simply could not participate in the exercise portion of a wellness program. When we explored this with him, he realized that his aversion to exercise went back to the time his physical education teacher had called him a "klutz." So, even as a mature and otherwise confident adult, he avoided exercise of any kind because he viewed himself as a klutz and was afraid of looking foolish. He was able to change that tape by replacing its message with one of his own: "I'm not going to let the careless remark of someone made years ago affect who I am today. I *know* I can exercise and enjoy all its fun and healthful benefits." Unless you take similar action to change your negative tapes, these tapes can continue to influence your self-image.

The world is indeed fortunate that the following people did not accept the messages they received:

* Thomas Edison was labeled "too stupid to learn."
* Grandma Moses was told she was too old to start painting at age 80.
* Winston Churchill was called "dull and hopeless" and failed sixth grade.

- Walt Disney, who loved to sketch and draw, was told he had no talent.
- Louis Pasteur was rated "mediocre" in chemistry.
- Abraham Lincoln did not allow himself to wallow in these failures:

> 1832 - lost job and was defeated for legislature
> 1833 - failed in private business
> 1835 - sweetheart died
> 1836 - had nervous breakdown and was defeated
>          for house speaker
> 1843 - was defeated for nomination to Congress
> 1848 - lost renomination
> 1849 - ran for land officer and lost
> 1854 - defeated for Senate
> 1856 - defeated for nomination for Vice President
> 1858 - defeated for Senate again

Other influences on your self-image appear throughout adulthood. Some of the early messages from your family will continue to be influential, in addition to new ones from coworkers, friends, social groups, clubs, religious groups, political organizations, and even comments and reactions from total strangers. We all have our own unique culture that feeds us information about who we are. These influences of adulthood are reinforced by the tapes of childhood.

The person who is overlooked for promotion at work may respond from a negative tape by saying: "Of course I wouldn't get the promotion. I've always been a loser." Or that person may respond from a positive tape by saying: "Well, I must not have been suited to that job. If I keep doing the quality work I know I am capable of, I'll get another opportunity for a promotion."

In this way life experiences reinforce the old tapes and make a stronger case for one's self-image. The diagnosis of a disease can likewise be approached as either the natural outcome of a lifetime of rotten luck or as a challenge that can be handled just as well as the previous life challenges you have handled.

Important and hopeful insight into human behavior and motivation comes from the world-famous Menninger Foundation's Center for Applied Behavioral Sciences. At the heart of this remarkable center is this philosophy:

*Your past is not your destiny.*

We do not have to make the same mistakes nor follow in the same life path and lifestyle to which we have become accustomed. We can make choices.

## You control your self-image

No matter what your various cultures are telling you about who you are, you can choose the messages to accept and the ones to reject. You do this by changing the messages you give yourself. You can change these messages by using one of the most effective mental tools known: positive self-talk. Mental health professionals call it "cognitive restructuring," the changing of one's thoughts. The basic premise behind this tool is that thought creates feeling. You change the way you feel about yourself by changing your thoughts.

The greatest revolution of our generation is the discovery
that human beings, by changing the inner attitudes of their
minds, can change the outer aspects of their lives.

—William James

The issue of aging has long been associated with this concept of
mind over matter. We have all observed that those who stay
"young at heart" seem to actually age more slowly than those who
think of themselves as being handicapped by advancing age.
George Burns, comedian, actor, and eighth wonder of the world,
made a wonderful observation when he turned 85:

Some people regard the age of 70 as old. They tell
themselves, "I'm 70 and 70 is old. How should I act now
that I'm old? Maybe I should sit down more slowly and
walk more slowly. Perhaps I should even spill a bit when
I eat." If these people practice really hard, by the time
they're 75, they're pretty good at acting old. I'm no good
at acting old because I never practice.

The important point is that George Burns refuses to accept the
message given him by society. He altered his own attitude toward
aging by giving himself positive messages like, "I can tap dance.
I'm not old!" Negative messages tarnish one's self-image only
if they are accepted as being self-descriptive.

## Choose to reject negative messages

You cannot escape negative messages. The world is full of them. But you can choose to reject them. People who get diseases are sometimes "labeled" with terms such as arthritic, cerebral palsied, cystic, depressed, diabetic, epileptic, etc. You must view these labels as shorthand descriptions of conditions some people have, not as descriptions of the individuals themselves. You can help our society avoid labels by using appropriate descriptions yourself. Phrases such as "a person with arthritis," or whatever the condition may be, avoid the tendency of the listener to judge or think of the person solely in terms of his or her disease.

You can choose to take a negative message and reject it by using a technique that Dr. Albert Ellis, a psychologist, refers to as "talking sense to yourself." I talked a lot of sense to myself after the following experience:

> I was at a party, chatting with a man I'd not met before. He launched into a lengthy description of his work. After a while he paused and asked, "What do you do?" I told him that I worked in health and well-being and had gotten started in it because I have diabetes. Just as I was about to describe my exciting work, he interrupted me to say, "Oh, that reminds me of a paper I wrote in college, 'Sterilization of Defectives.'"

Using the technique of talking to myself, I rejected this negative message. I told myself, "Having diabetes surely does not make me a 'defective.' What a dreadful label!" My own condemnation of the man's unfortunate remark became not the source of a bitter spirit but rather a commitment to sensitivity and a caring spirit.

That painful experience brought me growth. A moment like that is when illness can become wellness.

Hold a psychological mirror up to yourself. Review the experiences you've had, the messages you've received, and most important, the messages you've chosen to believe. Negative messages do not need to be dramatic to be destructive. They can, in fact, be quite unintentional.

At my clinic one day I gave myself an insulin injection with a disposable syringe. The nurse directed me to dispose of the syringe in a cardboard box in her office. When I looked at the box, I saw the word "contaminated." I was startled. Not understanding that the word was strictly a routine medical term, I took it as a negative insinuation. My message to myself to counter the inferred insult was, "I'm not defective and I'm not contaminated. I just have diabetes."

Negative messages will not be destructive if they are rejected and replaced by sensible messages. Old negative tapes from childhood can be quite persistent in influencing your self-image. If you hear an old "I've always been a loser" tape playing in your mind, try starting an argument with yourself. When you hear negative self-talk, argue back with positive facts. Get your "coach" working for you! Here is how to have a healthy argument:

Negative: "Who'd want to hire a cripple?"

Positive: "I'm not a cripple! I may not move as quickly as I used to, but my mind is excellent and I'm honest, hard-working, and loyal. Who wouldn't hire me?"

## Give yourself positive messages

Positive messages not only help to overcome a negative self-image, they are also needed to promote and maintain a positive self-image. "Daily affirmations" are one ongoing technique many have found helpful. An affirmation is a positive statement. Make a point of making a positive statement about yourself at least once a day. Just as it was a wise and loving coach who helped you argue with your negative self-messages, it is a wise and inspiring coach who gives you affirmations for encouragement.

A counselor with whom I worked not only recommends affirmations to his clients, he uses them regularly himself. In his office he has a sign that reads, "I am lovable and loving." It is only five words. It seems so simple. Yet it is a message that touches the heart of the human condition: our need to be accepted (loved) and to have the ability to love others. And it promotes a healthy, positive self-image. If you have a hard time deciding on your affirmation, consider using this one.

Repeat your affirmation daily. It may take months before you begin to notice feeling more positive about yourself. Keep at it. The outcome is well worth your effort.

A woman with whom I worked once felt that her lack of patience was causing her great stress. Her frequent comments of, "I am so impatient!" only affirmed that negative self-image. So she began giving herself a different affirmation: "I am relaxed. I am free of tension. I am patient." At a support group meeting several weeks after she began the positive affirmations, her husband remarked just how great a change he had noticed in her approach to daily tasks and annoyances.

The remainder of this chapter is a series of practical suggestions to help you develop a positive self-image.

## Affirm Y-O-U

Following are most of the letters of the alphabet. After the letters are words of a positive and constructive meaning. Write your name vertically down the left side of the page or on a separate sheet of paper. Next to each letter of your name write words that describe you or that you would like to have describe you. Using the word "capable" for the letter C does not mean that you are perfectly capable of doing everything. It means that you are capable in certain areas of your life. Everyone can honestly affirm that. For the C in my own name I would avoid words like "cold" or "careless." There surely may be times in my life when I have behaved in such a manner, but an isolated event does not define my whole identity. Remember that. Forgive yourself for what is past. Build a positive future with positive messages today.

A: able, abundant, accurate, active, adaptable, authentic
B: balanced, beautiful, beneficent, best, blessed, brave
C: capable, caring, character, compassionate, courageous
D: daring, debonair, decent, decisive, doer, distinctive
E: eager, earnest, effective, efficient, empathetic, energetic, expressive
F: fair, faithful, festive, fine, forthright, free, fun
G: gentle, genuine, giving, glad, good, grown-up, gutsy
H: healthy, handy, happy, honest, humanitarian
I: illuminating, important, improved, individual, industrious
J: jovial, joyful, judicious, just, jubilant
K: kind, kindhearted, knowledgeable, keen

L:  law-abiding, leader, level, lifeful, liked, lively, loving
M: mannerly, mature, merry, motivated, mover, musical
N: natural, navigator, needed, noble, novel
O: obedient, open, optimal, ordered, orderly, original
P: pacesetter, patient, peacemaker, peaceful, pleasant, practical
Q: quaint, qualified, quality, quick, quintessential
R:  radiant, ready, real, reasonable, relaxed, reliable, romantic
S:  self-disciplined, self-respecting, self-reliant, silly, solid, soft, spirited
T: tactful, tenacious, tender, thankful, thorough, tolerant
U: ultimate, unassuming, unique, upbeat, useful
V: valuable, versatile, vigorous, VIP, vital
W:warm, well, wholesome, winner, wise, worthwhile
Y: young, youthful, yourself
Z: zany, zesty, zingy, zippy

Look in the dictionary for even more ideas of constructive, positive words with which to describe yourself. Now, taking the letters of your name, choose a word to represent each letter and to describe the *you* that you want to be and *CAN* be! Give yourself a new middle initial or two if there are qualities you'd like to acquire. I give myself a P so I can add the affirmation, "I am patient."

## Positive behavior creates positive feelings

Now that you have a whole list of positive words describing you, take the next step of following through with appropriate behavior. Look at the words you've selected to correspond with the letters of your name, and ask yourself what behaviors would match those words. If you chose "caring" for the letter C, for instance, define the specific activities in which a caring person would engage. A caring person might volunteer some time at the local hospital or in a nursing home, visit a friend who needs a boost, or help a family member with a special project. The good feeling you get from the behavior you chose will help you to see yourself as a truly caring person.

A woman shared with me how she overcame her self-image as a sick person. She got busy helping other people. "When I help others, I see myself as a healthy, coping, giving person," she explained. She has learned how persuasive behavior is. By behaving like a coping, giving, healthy person, she came to see herself that way, and so did the people around her. It is, in fact, what she has become.

## Take charge through assertive behavior

When people behave nonassertively, they frequently view themselves as doormats—someone whom everyone else is free to walk on. That's a terrible self-image to carry into person-to-person encounters. Expressing one's opinions, ideas, and beliefs without fear of contradicting someone else or not going along with a group increases self-confidence and adds to a positive self-image. In their book *Your Perfect Right*, Robert Alberti and Michael Emmons define assertive behavior as:

> Behavior which enables a person to act in his/her own best interests, to stand up for him/herself without undue anxiety, to express his/her honest feelings comfortably or to exercise his/her own rights without denying the rights of others.

Assertiveness techniques are presented in Chapter 7, "Getting the Support You Need." Assertive communication is required to ask your friends, family, and medical team for the support you need from them.

Below is a sample of assertive behavior and its positive impact on self-image:

Marian's doctor told her about a new drug for her arthritis. From the way he explained it, Marian felt that it sounded like an experimental drug which had not yet been thoroughly tested. Some people feel comfortable trying experimental medications; Marian did not. She asserted herself by saying, "That sounds to me like it is too new to have been thoroughly tested. What are my other options?" After her appointment, Marian rode the clinic's elevator down to the lobby. It was apparent that someone was smoking. Marian again chose to be assertive. She turned to the person smoking, smiled, and in a firm but pleasant manner said, "I believe that there is no smoking allowed on elevators. There is an ash try just outside the door; if you wish to put your cigarette there, I'll be happy to hold the elevator for you."

The impact on Marian's self-image is quite evident in the self-talk she practiced on the way home. "I'm so glad I questioned that drug. I really felt uncomfortable about trying it. The doctor appreciated my honesty and the appointment went well. Not only did he advise me of a well-tested drug that he believes will help me, but I also had the distinct impression that our mutual honesty and clear communication enhanced our relationship. And I'm pleased about the elevator incident. He immediately put out his cigarette, apologized, and even thanked me for saying something. I feel good about myself."

## Keep an affirmations file

Everyone can keep a personal file that contains affirming, uplifting, and otherwise positive notes. I've kept such a file for many years, on the suggestion of the principal of the school where I taught. Put *your* name on the file flag and fill it with notes, letters, newspaper clippings, cards you've received over the years, and anything else that constitutes a positive message about you. Read through this file whenever your life seems a bit dreary. It can provide you with a wonderful shot in the arm! It is difficult to maintain a negative self-image when you read a note from someone that says: "Thank you for bringing your special love into my life. Your thoughtfulness was greatly appreciated." Stock your file with all those things that lift your spirits. I feel ten feet tall when I read some of the cards I've received from my young son. Each "I love you, Mommy" is a real spirit booster!

God gave us memories so that we might have roses in December.

—James M. Barrie

What a lovely thought that is. However, some people seem to find it easier to remember the thorns instead of the rose petals. So keep a collection of special thoughts to help you remember the life-affirming messages.

**Remember, you are special**

That is not an egotistical statement; it is a fact. Accept compliments when you receive them, because you deserve them. Avoid putting yourself down and never say, *"I am only..."* "You are YOU," and that's special because you are the best you in the world.

During the late 1970s, King Carl Gustav of Sweden visited Gustavus Adolphus College on his tour of the United States. Along with thousands of others, I attended the luncheon given for him in the hockey arena. I noted at one point the king straightened up and looked to one corner of the arena. I followed his gaze. There stood the food service director, Evelyn (the white tornado) Young and her team of student servers. Within minutes everyone in the arena was served a hot, delicious meal. The King led an ovation acknowledging her excellence in serving. Before leaving the United States to return to Sweden, he presented Mrs. Young with a medal for her outstanding accomplishment. She was decorated by European royalty for serving a meal well!

Another illustration of the importance of each individual is the following:

> You arx important! You arx xxcxptional! Thx nxxt timx you think you arx only onx pxrson and that your xfforts arx not nxxdxd, rxmxmbxr this typxwritxr and say to yoursxlf: I am a kxy pxrson! I am nxxdxd vxry much!

## Give yourself a pep talk

In *The Magic of Thinking Big*, David Schwartz encourages people to give themselves pep talks similar to a commercial. Like the exercise that encourages you to use words for each letter of your name, this exercise avoids boastful, bragging language in favor of simple, positive values that you hold. By writing and reciting this pep talk, you affirm these values and you'll feel increasingly better about yourself. You may wish to select some of the words from the name exercise to use in your pep talk. This is a brief example:

> (Your name), you are an adaptable person. That is an excellent quality. No matter what challenge or disappointment confronts you, you are able to adapt and regain balance. In the face of adversity you have demonstrated that you can be brave and even cheerful. You are compassionate and caring. You are a good friend to others as well as to yourself. You are doing well.

A friend of mine, a nurse, read Schwartz's book and wrote this type of affirming message for herself. She read it often in the days before an important interview. She told me the message gave her self-confidence a real boost.

## Thank people

It will enhance your self-image to see how grateful people are to receive *your* gratitude. Fill someone else's personal file of affirmations. Have you ever noticed that people who thank others a lot and always seem to notice the good that others do seem to be self-confident and have a positive self-image? Visualize yourself behaving in the same confident and generous manner. Then follow your mental blueprint for action by doing it. Psychologists tell us that behavior produces feeling. Tell people "thank you," send letters of appreciation to your bank, service station, child's teacher, a store or restaurant where you received good service; give thanks and praise generously. It will do *wonders* for how you feel about yourself.

## Mental images

Some people use metaphors to describe themselves. A metaphor is a figure of speech that uses one object or idea to suggest a likeness with another one. For example, some see themselves as mighty oak trees; others imagine themselves as their favorite folk hero.

When I was 11 years old, my brother asked me, "Do you know why we're so strong?" I immediately understood his question, because by that age I had already learned that life could be tough: Two years earlier our wonderful father had died, and one year after that, I developed diabetes. So to have survived and even thrived, I knew I was strong. But he answered his own question: "It's because we're half Canadian." Right away I pictured the image of a Mountie. But I couldn't relate to that metaphor, even though I'm proud of my Canadian heritage and admire the Royal Canadian Mounted Police. I did, however, have other heroes— mostly men and women from books or movies—after whom I modeled myself. In doing so I took strength and inspiration from them by imagining how they would respond to the various challenges I faced.

Many years later a clear and helpful metaphor emerged for me. A radio commentator was explaining why the large amount of rain that spring was potentially more harmful than helpful to the crops. He said that, coming in such excessive amounts, most of it ran off, while only a small amount remained near the surface of the soil. Thus, plants had such easy access to water they did not need to send their roots down deep to find it. A shallow root system, then, allows plants to be easily uprooted by normal seasonal storms.

As soon as I heard that story, I knew why I was strong as an adult: When I was just a little "sprout," my roots had to go down deep to find the river of life. So I'm a plant with incredibly deep roots, while my brother is Sergeant Preston of the Yukon. What metaphor describes you?

If a negative image (like a broken branch or a dried up well) comes to mind, reject it and choose a new metaphor. See yourself as a healthy, green branch with buds or a fresh, bubbling spring of water. Keep working at seeing yourself in this new, life-affirming metaphor. Eventually it will affect your self-image.

**Take charge!**

Keep in mind that your present age is the number of years that you have taken to develop your self-image. It certainly will not take that long to move toward a more positive one, but the process does take time. Use the suggestions offered in this chapter. Seek professional help if you know you are stuck in a negative self-image. Above all, take responsibility for your life and for your self-image. As Eleanor Roosevelt so succinctly put it: "No one can make you feel inferior without your consent."

## Summary

- Your self-image is who you think you are, and it determines what you do and how you feel about yourself. A positive self-image is your armor against negative messages and a powerful force to help you gain self-confidence in everything you do.

- Self-image serves as a blueprint for behavior. If you honestly view yourself and act in a way you would like to be described, you will find that you have become that way and are viewed as such by others.

- Messages received in childhood from parents, relatives, teachers, and friends are powerful influences on self-image. These messages become "tapes" that are played in our minds unless we consciously take action to change them.

- An effective way to change negative self-messages is to practice positive self-talk. Thought creates feeling, and by changing the way you think about something, you can change the way you feel. That will help you take positive action. Remember, your past is not your destiny.

- Negative messages are all around us. You must choose to reject them and likewise choose which messages you will believe and make part of your self-image. You can be your own coach, arguing against negative messages with positive messages that describe the healthy you.

- Use daily affirmations—simple positive statements about yourself—to promote and build on your positive self-image.

- Keep a written and mental list of words that describe positive characteristics you have and some that you would like to have. Use those words as guides for your behavior, which will create the positive image you seek.

- Assertive behavior is an important part of a positive self-image. Being able to express your views and feelings affirms your right to self-determination and says that you regard yourself as an important person.

- Keeping an affirmation file of everything that carries a positive message about you is an excellent spirit booster when things seem dreary.

- Remember you are special. Even things you do that may seem insignificant, if done well, can affirm your specialness and add to your positive self-image.

- Give yourself a pep talk that is like a commercial for yourself. It will be reflected in your feelings and actions.

- Be generous in your praise and thanks to others. It will do wonders for how you feel about yourself.

- Find apt, life-affirming metaphors to describe yourself. Eventually, they will affect your self-image

- Take charge of improving your self-image. If you are unsuccessful, seek professional help to get started.

## Reflection Questions

1. Reflect on messages you have received from others:

   My parents told me that:


   At work I am considered:


   My friends think I am:


   My family would describe me as:



2. Identify some of the negative tapes you play to yourself.



3. List positive self-talk statements as a replacement for the negative tapes.

4. Evaluate which practical suggestions given for developing a positive self-image will benefit you most today. (See pages 31 to 39.)

List the activities you will incorporate into your life.

5. Using the self-descriptions in this chapter, write a positive affirmation of you by stating "I am . . . .

# Motivation: Light Your Own Fire

"*I know* what to do. I just can't get motivated."
*—a heart patient who has been instructed
to strengthen his heart through an exercise program.*

"I felt real motivated right after class, but then I just sort of drifted back to all my old behaviors."
*—a woman with diabetes who has attended
classes on nutrition, exercise, blood glucose
monitoring, and stress management.*

"I am not motivated to do my exercises when it is so painful!"
*—a person with arthritis*

"I really want to do well. I have the desire. I just don't seem to be able to follow through. Is motivation my problem?"
*—any one of us.*

## Is motivation the problem?

Only *you* can answer that question for your own unique situation. In this chapter we will explore motivation using the definition, "the forces that influence the decisions we make." Further, the word "motive" is defined as "a need or desire that causes a person to act." If we have the desire to follow healthy behaviors, what forces influence us to behave in either a healthy or an unhealthy manner? The purpose of this chapter is to explore what motivates you, what influences your behavioral and attitudinal choices, and then to explore what plan you can follow to help you overcome the negative influences and find support for making healthy choices.

## Need and desire

Your health problem may be the "need" that sparks your initial motivation to follow a healthy lifestyle. Reflect on the following questions:

*How do you feel about the need to change your lifestyle?*

• Resentful?  What did I do to deserve this?  Why me?
• Grateful?  Here's the extra push I needed to finally make some positive changes in my life.

*In your opinion what will these new lifestyle behaviors mean in relation to the overall quality of your life?*

• "Quality of life" is now out of the question because you have to stop all the things you enjoy.

- A challenge at first because change is difficult, but, ultimately, an enhanced quality of life.

If *need* is perceived as a burden or a punishment, then your experience with motivation is likely to be a battle. You are unlikely to stay motivated to follow healthy behaviors because you don't want to follow them. Following them may mean the sacrifice of an enjoyable life or "giving in" to your disease. However, if need is perceived within the context of taking responsibility for your life and gaining instead of losing control, then motivation will seem more like personal discovery and growth. Following these healthy behaviors will uncover numerous challenges, but it will also lead you to discover the strength within you and the support around you, which will help you stay motivated. Need may be what gets you motivated initially. *Desire* will help keep you motivated. To assess your desire, it is helpful to explore what you value.

## Value

The following statements describe values that fuel some people's desire to follow healthy behavior. Reflect on what you value.

- I want to live long enough to see my children grow up.
- I want to feel as well as I possibly can.
- self-respect
- besides managing the effects of my disease, receiving a benefit to my overall health
- serving as a positive role model for my children
- continuing work, tennis, golf, etc.

Go on with your own list. Take time to reflect on what you do and why you do it. Studies of people recovering from heart attacks showed that those who made the most progress were pet owners who otherwise lived alone. They took care of themselves, that is, eating regularly and exercising, because that's what they did for their pets. **Value** is one of the important foundations for motivation. The other important foundation is **belief.**

## Belief

You *value* health and well-being. But do you *believe* that you can be well? You will not be motivated to do anything unless you believe that it will lead to a positive outcome. People who believe aspirin will relieve their aches and pains are motivated to take it. People with arthritis may find it painful to do the prescribed exercises; it would be easy to skip them to avoid the accompanying pain. But if they *value* mobility and *believe* that the exercises can lead to that, they are more likely to be motivated to exercise. Many factors influence what we believe. As you read through the following, reflect on forces influencing your values and beliefs.

### Family tradition

Families pass on traditions in thinking and behaving. You may believe that you were meant to be fat because everyone in your family is overweight. This belief will lead to the behaviors that will assure that you become and remain overweight. Some family traditions are clearly unhealthy. What are your family traditions? Some are wonderfully healthy: serving Thanksgiving dinner to the homeless each year, participating in healthful activity after dinner instead of gathering around the television.

My husband's family is Norwegian, and one of their Christmas traditions is serving *rommegrot*, a thick cream pudding. Throughout the years, my husband has come to view this pudding as a high calorie, high-fat, artery-clogging food, which he chooses to eat a small portion of once a year. People who eat it frequently are more likely to view it as a strong, emotional tie to their roots.

Family tradition can be a warm, loving bond for everyone to enjoy. Examine closely the traditions within your family. If you find unhealthy traditions, see if you can think of healthy alternatives. For example, instead of bringing Grandma's rich goodies to every family get together, encourage family members to bring a favorite memory and have an evening of family storytelling. Stories will nourish your heart and soul but won't add an ounce of weight! The influence of our past can remain with us throughout adulthood.

One of the most dramatic examples I've seen of this involves a man at a seminar for people with diabetes. As I was teaching the seminar, I noticed him sitting in the back of the classroom. He seemed very angry. He never participated in any of our discussions. He simply glared and frowned throughout the class.

After the third class, he approached me when everyone else had gone. He said: "Anyone who has diabetes and doesn't admit he's inferior is a G.D. liar!" I asked him how he had been told he had diabetes. That crucial introduction strongly influences what one believes. He replied, "Well, I was ten years old and my mother and my doctor sat me down and said, 'You are sick. You can't go out for sports anymore or play with your friends the way you used to, because you're sick now.'"

Having been influenced in this way by these authority figures in his life, he believed that having diabetes meant that he would have to give up all the fun things in life. By the time I met him he had spent over 20 years believing he was sick and his life could never be fulfilling. He was living his life accordingly.

I couldn't help but think of the sharply contrasting situation of my experience with diabetes. I too was ten years old when I got diabetes. My father had died suddenly ten months before I was diagnosed. When my mother came into my hospital room, the doctor had just told me that I had diabetes. I asked her, "What does that mean?"

With a big smile on her face, my magnificent mother said, "Why, it means that we're going to learn so much about good nutrition. We're going to live such a healthy lifestyle that our whole family will benefit. And you will always be a stronger, more disciplined person because you have diabetes."

She had me sold! I wanted to go back to school and give it to my friends! Her positive belief, given with such conviction, became my belief. The experience shaped my life—as one's culture so often does.

Motivation experts describe yet another aspect of the motivational power of belief with the statement: **"Expectation becomes self-fulfilling prophecy."** This concept is illustrated in the following examples:

The father of an acquaintance of mine comes from a family in which none of the men have lived beyond the age of 55. As this man approaches his mid-fifties, what do you suppose he's doing to preserve his health? Nothing. He smokes three packs of cigarettes a day and drinks to excess. He expects to die young. He is acting in a manner to bring that expectation to a self-fulfilled prophecy.

When my wonderful brother Pete was 38 years old, he had a heart attack. It was, of course, shocking and difficult for all of us who love him. My first thought was for Pete's recovery and future well-being. Understanding the concept of expectation and belief, I was concerned that Pete's expectation for his future be positive. My father was 42 when he died of a heart attack. How easy it would have been for Pete to resign himself to a premature death. To encourage Pete's spirit of determination, I gave him Norman Cousins' book, *Anatomy of an Illness*. He loved it. It lifted his spirits greatly.

Then I arranged for Pete and his wife to attend a weekend wellness retreat, where I knew he would gain information on living well, within the context of a supportive culture. One of the important messages he got was that although heredity is certainly a risk factor in heart disease, he has control over virtually every other risk factor. A combination of factual information, loving support, and Pete's own determination and love for life helped him to choose a positive expectation. His cholesterol dropped significantly as he changed his eating habits and began a regular exercise program.

I know that Pete genuinely believes in his healthy future. When he turned 40 he had braces put on his teeth!

Please do some careful self-examination at this point. What are your beliefs about your health challenge, and more important, about your future well-being? The Health Belief Model states that in order to take positive action toward health, people need three things: to understand the seriousness of their disease, to believe that they are personally vulnerable, *and* to have a strong, hopeful belief that they can do something to positively affect the outcome.

## Culture

The wider culture is also a powerful influence in our choices. To understand the impact of culture on your life explore the various cultures from your past and present. Culture includes ethnic background, family of origin and current family, neighborhood, schools, friends, and jobs.

Jackie Townsend provides a remarkable example of the power of positive belief as an antidote to negative cultural messages. I heard Jackie, a former Miss America, speak several years ago. After her reign, she married and had a son and then a daughter. One night she awakened to hear her infant daughter crying. She tried to go to her baby but could not move. She was totally paralyzed. She tried to tell her husband that she needed help. She couldn't speak. At the age of 28 she had suffered a massive stroke. She spent the next years learning all over again to walk and talk.

Jackie had tremendous family support and still does. She told us the only residual impact of her stroke is that when she becomes emotional, her words don't always come out. She told us that recently she was scolding her son, now a teenager. Suddenly, the words stopped coming. Her son waited a moment, then enthusiastically cried out, "Come on, Mom, you can do it!"

Two older women were sitting in front of me. One turned to the other and said, "Well, that's youth!" I disagree: *That's belief!* Jackie refused to believe the cultural messages surrounding her about stroke "victims" and the "vegetables" they become. She replaced those negative messages with positive messages such as "Jackie, you're 28 years old, you've got two babies, and you're going to make it!" She believed in the positive outcome she ultimately achieved.

## Advertising

Some of our strongest cultural messages come from the advertising in magazines and newspapers, on television and radio. Advertisers appeal to our emotions. What are some of the television, radio, magazine, or billboard ads that influence you? What emotion or human need does each of these ads appeal to in order to sell its product? We need to be smart consumers and always aware of an ad's influence on our emotions. If an ad makes a claim, verify it before you buy the product. Base your decision on facts, not emotions. Perhaps the most insidious aspect of advertising is in what is implied, not openly stated or "claimed." The image of an attractive young person engaging in strenuous physical activity while smoking implies that attractive, athletic people smoke. Wealthy, attractive, and happy persons consuming alcoholic beverages in the ad suggest that "successful" people drink. The next time you view, hear, or see an ad, analyze what it is trying to do. Make your choices fully aware of what the advertiser wants and what *you* want.

It is challenging to believe in a positive future when you are surrounded by negative messages about your future. During national diabetes month each year, for instance, I find it challenging as a person with diabetes to remain positive and believe in my healthy future when I read billboards telling of the blindness, kidney failure, and heart attacks so closely associated with diabetes. At times it is extremely difficult to believe. But it is possible to do so.

## Human nature

In 1912, Stacy Adams proposed what is called the "Equity Theory of Motivation." Adams said that everyone has a sense of fairness and, if treated fairly, people respond by working fairly. Adams' observation describes a feeling that seems quite common in American culture. In this nation of free enterprise, we are accustomed to receiving rewards in direct proportion to the amount of work we've done. "Work hard and you will be rewarded" has been a national expectation throughout our history. It appeals to a sense of fairness that Adams says most of us have.

Therefore, it strikes people as unfair when they follow closely the recommended medical regimen only to find little or no improvement in their condition. They feel cheated out of a reward for their efforts. A person with cancer who does not respond to painful, unpleasant treatments may know of someone with the same cancer who is responding to treatment. That isn't fair, but unfortunately, it is the nature of disease and medicine: Everyone responds a bit differently.

Likewise, a person with arthritis may say, "Esther and I got arthritis at about the same time five years ago. Today she's walking and I can hardly hobble. It isn't fair!" Or, "My neighbor Harry smokes more than I do and is even more overweight. How come I had a heart attack? It isn't fair." Of course it isn't fair. It isn't that you would wish these individuals were afflicted as much as you. It's just that you would like to be as fortunate as they. There is no magic answer to relieve the frustration and anguish we feel in these situations. Life simply isn't fair. We want it to be, but it isn't. Awareness of this inherent element of being human may not remove the frustration, but it may bring you insight into yourself and humanity, which will prove helpful to you.

In a *Harvard Business Review* classic we find another aspect of human nature and its impact on motivation. Douglas MacGregor called it the "Theory X, Theory Y" approach to human motivation. This approach states that people are more motivated if they have input into decisions that affect them. Darlene and Susan illustrate this theory. Darlene has diabetes and reports that her dietitian never asked her a question about what food she likes or dislikes. The dietitian simply handed Darlene a meal plan and told her to follow it. To Darlene, diabetes means you lose control of your life; people tell you what to do.

Susan, on the other hand, reports that her dietitian asked a lot of questions about food preferences as well as about Susan's eating schedule. When Susan's meal plan was completed, she felt that she had designed it herself. To Susan, diabetes means learning to make healthy choices, staying in control of her life.

And another classic in human nature and motivation is Abraham Maslow's hierarchy of needs. Maslow described that hierarchy of human needs with a pyramid shape, explaining them thus: At the base of the pyramid are life's most basic and fundamental needs: shelter, water, food. The needs progress through social, self-esteem and, finally, self-actualization. Maslow observed that people are motivated by the lowest level of current, unmet needs and that a fulfilled need no longer motivates. The Life Satisfaction Survey in chapter one is intended to help you discover your unmet needs. You may want to thoughtfully consider their importance to you and create your own pyramid, according to their priority for you.

**Self-image** is such an important influence in motivation that we devoted an entire chapter to it.

Review all the influences that have been described, and then add ones of your own. Reflect on how each influence can be positive or negative. Our responsibility then is to *assess* the impact of the influences on our lives to make choices: to increase the influences that help and to limit the influences that hinder us.

## Hopelessness is a major obstacle to motivation

People will not be motivated to take good care of themselves if they believe their situation is hopeless. This hopelessness is seen in such comments as "My mother had arthritis, and she ended up in a wheelchair. That's where I'm headed." Or, "My father died of a heart attack at a young age. So will I." Or, "I've heard that diabetes is the leading cause of blindness. What's the use in trying to beat the odds?" Or, "Everyone know that cancer kills."

The feeling of hopelessness comes from such messages of hopelessness. One way to fight hopelessness is to argue back. Give yourself a message like this: "There is so much more known about my disease today. Each day brings more information and better treatments, with the possibility of a major breakthrough in research. I will learn all I can. I will seek the best medical support. I will do all I can to manage my disease. And I will manage my feelings by continuing to give myself positive, encouraging messages. I am doing well."

Hopelessness is like a bucket of water extinguishing the flame of motivation. We need a whole box of motivational matches to relight our flame whenever it goes out.

**Keeping the flame lit**

Achieving goals is motivating because success builds on success. Set small goals for yourself; you'll achieve them within a fairly short period of time. Then set the next goal immediately, reach it, set the next, and so on. You will experience a motivational boost to your spirit as you continue to look forward to your next goal. And you will experience a motivational momentum as you have one success after another. A friend of mine wanted to start a regular exercise program when she was in her mid-forties. Since it was well over twenty years since she had done much physical exercise, she was unsure of whether she could really do it. Wisely, she started slowly. Her first goal was to walk to the end of the block and back. Steadily she increased the distance and the vigor with which she walked. She eventually became a runner, running seven miles at a time! You start by setting goals you can easily achieve.

Improved health and a greater sense of being in control of life can come from working toward clear and carefully defined goals that you have set for yourself. Listen to the suggestions of your carefully selected advisors, but choose your own goals. You are ultimately responsible for yourself. You decide whether to accept the advice and whether to carry it out.

One of my mentors, Dr. Leonard Mastbaum, a Minneapolis endocrinologist, has an interesting way of encouraging clients to set their own goals. In his wisdom he realizes that the only goals persons will strive to attain are the goals they have set for themselves. Dr. Mastbaum draws a continuum, a straight line with a zero at one end and a ten at the other:

0..........................................................................................................................10

He calls it a management continuum. The zero means that the client chooses to do nothing to manage his or her disease. The ten symbolizes perfection; that is, the client is willing to do absolutely everything that is recommended. After explaining this, he asks the client to choose how much he or she is willing to do to manage the disease.

Apply this concept to your situation. Make a list of all the behaviors you would do if you were following your physician's advice perfectly. Then decide how many of the behaviors you are willing to incorporate into your life. If your physician has recommended ten behaviors, and you decide that you are willing

THE PHYSICIAN WITHIN / 59

to do five, place yourself in the middle of the continuum. Then have a very candid discussion with your physician about the consequences of your proposed behaviors. Depending on your situation, your physician may say that your goal is perfectly reasonable and likely to lead to a good outcome. Or your physician may say that 50 percent adherence to the recommendations will likely give you a 50 percent chance of doing well.

Our nature inclines us to take some "leeway" in carrying out advice we are given. Look at your continuum and set a realistic goal for yourself. People don't always experience success even when they cooperate with the recommendations of their medical team. Sometimes things happen that are beyond anyone's control. The disease may worsen. A particularly promising therapy may not work. At best, you can be philosophical about setbacks and disappointments. At worst, your disappointment can stop your good efforts and darken your hope. Frustration is a major obstacle to motivation when it gets out of hand. This frustration stems from the natural feeling that your efforts should be rewarded. And indeed they should. Your reward might not always be a positive health outcome, but it is important that your efforts be rewarded in some significant way.

## Reward is a motivator

Rewards are particularly effective motivators when the objective is to change behavior. It is called Behavior Modification. But what it boils down to is this: When you get a reward for doing something, you are more likely to do it again. Behavior that is rewarded is repeated. This motivation technique is used in toilet training for children, obedience training for dogs, coaching athletes, and supervising employees. There is no reason it can't be used just as effectively for self-motivation!

In general, motivation by reward is most effective when used to achieve short-term goals. Getting your reward quickly will help in the early stages of beginning a behavior change. And, especially when attempting to change a long-standing habit, you need regular, frequent rewards along the way to keep you going. For this reason, it is important to *reward behavior—not results.*

Let's look at weight loss as an illustration of this point. For a variety of reasons, weight loss can be a very slow process. If you were to wait until you'd reached your desired result of, say, 30 pounds before you rewarded yourself, you would have a very long wait. The lack of a reward during that time will serve as a reminder that you have not succeeded or perhaps are not even making good progress. The resulting frustration could lead to discouragement and giving up. The answer is to reward yourself for the positive behaviors of following your special meal plan, exercising, and avoiding situations that you associate with over-eating.

Fred wanted to change his behaviors to achieve a more consistent lifestyle. Long business lunches and sleeping in on weekends were interfering with the exercise program designed to strengthen his mending heart. He set a goal of allowing no more than one lunch per week to interrupt his exercise, and he set another goal of sleeping in no more than one extra hour on weekends. He kept track on his calendar of how he was doing. Then, on the 15th and 30th of each month, he checked to see how he'd done. His reward for following positive behavior was to buy tickets to a baseball game, an extra afternoon of golf, or a professional shoe shine (something he really enjoyed but considered to be a bit extravagant—a perfect reward!).

Each individual must decide on his or her own rewards, because they must be things that truly appeal to you. Rewards need not be expensive. An afternoon at the art institute or a day spent browsing through a shopping center may be perfect. These rewards may require family cooperation if you need a babysitter while you're gone. Be creative. Make a list of all the possible rewards you could give yourself. Keep the list handy.

To help you get started on your own list of rewards here is a beginning:

- —a leisurely bath by candlelight with music
- —a new book and time set aside for reading it
- —an hour to listen to music you especially enjoy
- —new make-up or a hair appointment
- —tickets to a favorite event
- —special time together with a friend
- —a walk through a rose garden
- —a small gift to yourself: a scarf, belt, cologne
- —extra time to spend on your favorite hobby
- —a brief vacation or trip
- —an extended vacation, if you can afford it
- —a telephone conversation with a special friend
- —that class you've always wanted to take
- —go on with your list . . . .

Receive a double benefit from your reward by reminding yourself as you enjoy it that you have earned it! Tell yourself that you are a winner and get daydreaming about your next reward!

## Positive Reinforcement

Sometimes I wish I had a cheerleader to follow me around giving me messages of encouragement and enthusiastically congratulating me every time I did well. Parents, teachers, and other authority figures play important roles as "cheerleaders" for children. But adults need that boost too. A psychiatrist friend of mine said once that people need encouragement like plants need water. Humans have "recognition hunger." People like to receive recognition: everything from a simple hello from a friend to an award for an outstanding accomplishment. That's positive reinforcement. Motivation experts such as Frederick Herzberg, a businessman, point out that positive reinforcement is one of the greatest motivators known. Because it fulfills our hunger for recognition, positive reinforcement motivates us to repeat the behavior.

An amusement park instituted an incentive motivation program for their young employees. Customers were given cards that read: "Nice going!" They were asked to give a card to any of the park employees who were especially helpful or courteous. The plan was to have the employees turn in their cards at the end of the season for cash or prizes. The park's customers not only willingly handed out the cards, they also wrote personal messages on them: "Dear Vicki, Thank you for being so nice to our family. You made our day!" To the surprise of park officials, the young people didn't turn in their cards. The kind words—the positive reinforcement—were considered a greater reward than cash or prizes. Fortunate is the person who regularly receives positive reinforcement for his or her healthy behaviors. Even if you do not have those people cheering you on, you can train your internal coach to give you positive reinforcement.

Train your coach by first listening to the messages you give yourself. Are they positive ("Nice going, Mary") when you succeed, and generous ("That's okay, you'll do better next time") when you don't succeed? Do you accept the positive messages and compliments of others? ("Thank you, I'm so pleased you like it.") Or do you throw compliments away? ("What, this old thing?") Fire a negative coach. Train your coach to be helpful to you by giving you only positive and constructive messages.

Another motivating aspect of positive reinforcement is that you receive a real boost when you give positive reinforcement to others. This boost is spirit-lifting! Most agree that people are more likely to be motivated when they're feeling up rather than down. A Minneapolis industrial psychologist, Dr. Robert Hobert, states that through their behavior, people have a great deal of control over whether they feel up or down. Behavior creates feeling, thus reinforcing others makes them feel "up." A program Hobert presented to a major brokerage house was entitled, "How to stay up in a down market." His message was, "Give out positive reinforcement." This includes smiles, winks, handshakes, hugs, sincere compliments, any positive communication that positively reinforces another person.

The best way to learn about this is to try it for yourself. I tried it at the supermarket one day and the experience left me glowing:

One day I was grocery shopping and I asked the produce manager if he had any fresh spinach. He asked me to wait while he went to the back room to get it. He returned with a bag of spinach. Then he carefully and courteously explained how I should wash it in cold water and drain it on paper towels. I thanked him.

As I made my way through the store, I saw a man who looked as if he might be the manager. A voice inside me said, "Practice what you preach, Catherine. Go tell the store manager what a nice produce manager he has." So I approached him and asked if he were the store manager. He instantly took a defensive posture and said suspiciously, "Yes?" I then said, "Well, I just wanted you to know that your produce manager makes it a pleasure to shop in your store. He is helpful and courteous, and I just wanted to thank you." The store manager beamed a proud smile and thanked me.

What a positive feeling I received from that experience. Create your own positive feelings by giving out positive reinforcement to the people in your life. Work at doing it every day until it becomes a habit. You can experience a continual uplift from the practice!

## Perks

"Perks" are those persons, places, and experiences that remind us how good it is to be alive. Who or what are the perks in your life? If you were to make a list, people on it might include friends who make you laugh—acquaintances who are really turned on by life and who make you feel excited every time you talk with them—

people whom you greatly admire and who inspire you through their conversation, books, lectures, or sermons. Places might include the mountains or a quiet local creek. Your experiences list would probably be boundless and might include attending the symphony or the local high school's production of a musical, singing in your favorite group, spending a weekend at a lake cabin, or watching a gorgeous sunset with a friend who enhances your enjoyment by sharing the experience with you.

Occasionally in life there occurs a truly "mountaintop experience." When you have such an outstanding experience, it serves as a perk while you experience it and then continues to give you a boost as long as you retain the memory. I had such an experience when I heard Maria von Trapp speak. She is the woman about whom "The Sound of Music" was written. She stated that her philosophy of life was described well by one of the songs from the movie:

> *A bell's not a bell till you ring it.*
> *A song's not a song till you sing it,*
> *and love wasn't meant in your heart to stay.*
> *Love isn't love till you give it away.*

I still get shivers every time I remember that wonderful woman with her tanned, deeply lined, gracious old face, speaking those words so clearly and proudly. It will serve as one of my perks as long as I can recall that scene to mind.

Take charge of the perk-giving in your own life! Make a list of all the perks you can possibly give yourself. Consider these perks your "resources for renewal" and go to them often. The time to think about getting yourself "up" is on a regular basis, not when you're so far down that it's really difficult to get back up again. Take a moment right now to begin your list of perks.

## Habits

A Spanish proverb says: "Habits are at first cobwebs, then cables." And habits are both friends and enemies. When they're positive, they help us to establish healthy behaviors. But habits can present tremendous obstacles to our progress in making healthy choices if those habits are unhealthy.

After all my years of working in health, I have concluded that **it's easier to begin a new habit than to change an old one.** To defeat the old habit, any new habit should be incompatible with the old. A nurse tells the story of wanting to quit smoking. It was hard for her to quit, and she kept taking up her smoking habit again. Then she began a regular exercise program. The more vigorously she exercised, the less she smoked because she needed the increased breathing capacity for the hard workouts. This continued until she finally gave up smoking completely.

Make a list of your habits. Then divide the list into those habits that are healthy and helpful and those that are unhealthy and harmful. Next to the unhealthy habits, indicate a new behavior that could successfully compete with it and establish itself in the old habit's place. To get primed for this activity, *visualize* yourself free of the old habit as you engage in the new one.

## Visualization

Visualization is a mental image or picture. To see yourself free of the old habit, get a picture in your mind of yourself engaging in a new one. If you are to change, you must visualize yourself changed. That mental image is a powerful motivational tool.

A futurist whom I heard speak at a long-range planning meeting once made the observation that no nation, corporation, or individual can hope to move forward positively without a belief in a positive future. He called this a "positive future self-image." *That* is what you must visualize: your positive future self-image. And then you must believe it. Logic sometimes does battle with intuition, making it difficult to believe a visualized image. However, intuition will be more powerful than logic in persuading you to believe.

The brain has two hemispheres, the left brain and the right. The left side views things logically. The right side views things intuitively. Some people tend to be more logical and others more intuitive. For those more heavily influenced by logic, it may be difficult to be intuitive and to believe in anything not actually seen.

To encourage the intuitive side of yourself, think of times you've actually seen the effect of the mind on the body, such as when you feel a cold coming on but you decided you're too busy to get sick, and at bedtime you visualize yourself at work the next day, busy, energetic, and *well.* Or times when someone challenged you by saying you couldn't do something and you *decided* you could do it, and you did! Recalling actual examples is a way of combining logic with intuition. You believe because you've seen. With time, practice, and faith, you will believe after seeing it only in your mind.

One of the most common uses of visualization is in sports. For years coaches have told their athletes, "Before you perform, see yourself doing it!" Thus, basketball players visualize the ball swishing through the basket before they actually shoot. Golfers "see" their golf ball land on the green before they actually hit the ball.

Visualization works if it is supported by belief. I had lunch with a corporate president one day to plan a motivational program for his employees. He told me that he was playing golf after lunch. Without explaining the concept, I merely suggested to him that he visualize where he wanted each shot to go before he hit it. He said he'd try it. When I got to his company several weeks later, the first question I asked was about his golf game and visualization. "It didn't work," he told me. However, after I gave my presentation and explained the importance of belief, he rushed up to me exclaiming, "That's it! I visualized, but I didn't believe. I said to myself, 'That's where I want it to go, but it won't.'" Visualize *and* believe.

Believing is hard. But if you are to find the motivation to follow a healthy lifestyle and any self-care required by your disease, you must believe there is hope for a positive outcome.

Now, a positive outcome may mean that the physical complications are less severe or that a remission of the disease occurs. But outcome may go far beyond the physical experience. A positive outcome may mean that by living a meaningful life, by enjoying the "process," spiritual peace and joy are achieved.

I believe that a positive outcome can be defined as personal growth, in which persons so transcend their pain that they come to view their suffering as a blessing because of the growth it brought.

Come to your own understanding of the motivational power of belief. You can pursue a positive outcome while recognizing the beauty and fulfillment of the process of living.

## Is motivation the problem?

We return to the original question, and a never-ending one at that. After exploring the issue of motivation as it relates to your challenge and your life, you may have received an insight that helped remove an obstacle or reinforce a belief. It may be a good idea to wait until you have explored all the issues in this book before you attempt to answer the question of whether motivation is your problem. Maybe a stress in your life is demanding your energy and distracting you from your goal. It isn't that you are unmotivated. You are *stressed*. Maybe your support system is not sufficiently developed. You may need to work at decreasing the stress in your life and increasing your support. Only you can answer the question: **What do I need to get myself motivated?**

## Summary

- Motivation is the combination of forces that influence the decisions we make. Needs and desires motivate us to behave in certain ways.

- At bottom, motivation rests on the twin foundations of values and beliefs.

- Those values and beliefs are generally shaped by our families and the wider culture; but we must examine and challenge these standards to limit their influence on us.

- Set your own goals in small, achievable steps, using advice from selected advisors.

- Choose rewards for yourself and enjoy them often to motivate yourself for further success.

- Train your internal coach to give you regular positive comments; go out of your way to make positive comments about others.

- "Perks" are persons, places, and experiences in life that remind us how good it is to be alive. Define your perks and make use of them often to keep yourself "up."

- Examine your habits. If they are unhealthy, they can be great obstacles to progress in making healthy choices.

- Visualizing yourself looking healthy now and in the future will increase positive outcomes.

- Positive outcome does not necessarily mean a complete remission or cure; it can mean the personal growth that comes from living a meaningful life.

## Reflection Questions

1. Reflect on what a "fulfilling life" means to you. This is the foundation for your motivation. It is what you hope for, what you live for. Close your eyes and see yourself participating in this happy, healthy, fulfilling life. Be specific in your vision.

> What do you look like?

> Where are you?

> What are you doing?

> How do you feel?

> What changes do you need to make to enable that vision to come true?

> List three steps you can take right now that will lead to toward your fulfilling life. Consider these "steps" to be your goals.

2. Identify what you value. (Refer to the bottom of page 47 if you need to.)

Do you believe these values are possible? Why or why not?

It is important to believe that what you do will lead to a positive outcome. If you have discovered that your values and beliefs are not positively connected, talk to a trusted counselor, friend, or member of your medical team about this.

3. List rewards that will motivate your behavior in reaching your goals. (Some options on page 61 might appeal to you.)

# CHAPTER 4

# Adapting to Life's Challenges

S aplings bend during storms and consequently do not break. We need to bend when life's storms hit us so we won't break under the stress. I call that adaptability.

Adaptability may be one of the most important qualities of a healthy life. The circumstances of life change continually. Either we adapt to fit these changing circumstances or our well-being suffers. As I look back over a variety of challenging circumstances in my life, I believe one of my most helpful assets is my ability to adapt.

When my Brownie troop held its first father-daughter banquet after my father's death, I could have chosen not to attend. Instead, I invited my father's best friend to be my escort. It became a fun tradition, which he and I enjoyed all the years I was in scouting. I miss my father to this day, but I did adapt to life without him.

When I was ten years old I got diabetes. Living well with diabetes has been a continuing exercise in adaptability. As a ten year old, I went to slumber parties and brought all my equipment with me so I could do my testing and give my shots. Likewise, I went on Girl Scout campouts, played in the marching band, and participated in sports. Having diabetes just meant I had to think through a few more situations than the other kids—I had to adapt.

My need for adaptability will continue throughout my life. Once I flew to a meeting and the airline confirmed twice that the flight was a meal flight. Once aboard the plane, however, I was told there was no food. That's a potentially serious situation for a person with insulin-dependent diabetes who isn't prepared to adapt. I adapted to the situation by eating food I had brought with me.

Personality tests indicate that adaptability is a universally human quality. Some people are by nature highly adaptable, while others find it difficult to adapt. Among the most human people in medicine are those who accept individual differences in their patients' ability to adapt. But those same wise health professionals know that everyone, except for the seriously mentally ill, can choose to improve their ability to adapt. Once an individual has made the choice to improve, he or she can learn skills and find the necessary support to make healthy adaptations to the changing circumstances of life.

Diabetes and most chronic diseases require lifestyle changes. When it is possible to make slow, incremental changes, the overall change is more likely to become permanent. An example of incremental change is moving from whole to skim milk. An excellent way to lower fat in one's diet, it is commonly viewed as a drastic change from "real" milk to "blue water." Moving from whole to 2%, staying there until you are perfectly comfortable, and then moving to 1% and skim is much easier and usually assures success.

## Many life events require adaptability

Adaptability is not a skill reserved just for living well with a disease. It is a necessary part of every healthy life. Just think of all the times people *have* to adapt!

- When the fourth person shows up for dinner and there are three chicken breasts. (Your menu changes to stir fry chicken.)

- When the projector bulb burns out in the middle of a slide presentation. (You quickly learn to graphically describe visuals.)

- Getting laid off from a job. (Teaches you creativity to live more simply and adaptability to discover new skills.)

- Spraining the thumb on your writing hand when you have a paper due tomorrow. (Typing is slow without your thumb, but you figure out how to do it.)

That's life. You adapt to its changing circumstances because you must. To do otherwise would mean giving up and missing out on what life has to offer to its survivors. One of the important qualities that makes people survivors is their ability to adapt. And adapting to a challenge to their health is one of the most crucial adaptations they can make.

Eventually we all are confronted with the challenge of coping with physical limitation, whether it be from illness, injury, or simply aging. Each of us must make our own separate peace with this issue. People with a disease or injury face this challenge earlier in their lives. People who are basically free of disease all their lives meet the issue of physical limitation when their body systems simply begin to slow down with age.

The following describes a beautiful attitude with which to meet physical limitation. If you can hold and adopt this attitude, then your limitation will truly be confined to the physical.

> I like spring, but it is too young. I like summer, but it is too proud. So I like best of all autumn; because its leaves are a little yellow, its tone mellower, its colors richer. And it is tinged a little with sorrow. Its golden richness speaks not of the innocence of spring, nor of the power of summer, but of the mellowness and kindly wisdom of approaching age. It knows the limitations of life and is content.
>
> —Lin Yutang

One of my family's most treasured friends lived to be 97 years old. Throughout the years we were continually inspired by Bob's healthy approach to life and living. It delights me to remember that he bowled in a league until he was 96! During the years we bowled with him, we did see a gradual decline in his "approach" to the bowling alley, but his approach to life never wavered. He was pragmatic about his declining physical state. Only occasionally would he mention that he noticed about every five years he wasn't quite able to do what he had done five years earlier. Most of the time Bob talked of the future. He was forward-thinking, active, and full of the life around him. Although he outlived two wives and spent his last years alone, he never seemed lonely. We invited Bob to our home frequently, not because we felt sorry for him, but because we thoroughly enjoyed him as a stimulating, inspiring friend. Because he adapted to his challenges with such peace, strength, and humor, I regard him as one of my most important role models.

Many people face adaptation to physical limitation much earlier in their lives. The person who becomes near-sighted gets glasses. This common and relatively minor adaptation allows him or her to see well again and continue enjoying a visually healthy life.

People with allergies or asthma adapt to their challenge by avoiding the food or other source of their allergic reaction. Some people require medication or even as great an adaptation as a move to another part of the country.

People with diabetes must make adaptations in their entire lifestyle. To successfully adapt to the disease's requirements they must eat nutritiously and often according to a time schedule. Some need to take pills or daily injections of insulin. Most people with diabetes are instructed to do daily finger stick blood tests to determine if their blood sugar is within a healthy range. Daily exercise and ongoing stress management are also necessary if one is to live well with diabetes.

People recovering from a heart attack or heart surgery must adapt their work schedule, exercise and activity, meals, and stress management. Medications and medical equipment may also become a necessary part of a healthy life.

Each health challenge presents its own demands, each of which requires *adaptation*.

Obviously, adaptation is not always as easy as getting a pair of glasses and wearing them. Some health challenges are very complex. The medical aspects of a healthy adaptation to one's disease require a highly skilled and committed team of health care providers to give advice on the physical requirements posed by each health challenge. Each of you reading this book must take the responsibility to find a medical resource to advise you on how to make wise and healthy adaptations to accommodate the requirements of your disease. And you can do this while still pursuing your hopes and dreams for a happy, fulfilling life.

## Adapt rather than accept

An interesting study was done some years ago using infants. A cold, metal sheet was laid next to the infants in a bassinet. Some of the babies turned away from the cold as soon as they felt it. Other babies simply lay there and cried.

The spirited adaptability of the first group of babies is similar to the spirit found in a group called the Candlelighters. They are a group of parents whose children have cancer. They get together to offer support to each other and others. They have chosen to light a candle instead of cursing the darkness.

Acceptance of one's disease or its limitations can be negative if it leads to resignation or hopelessness. Acceptance is negative if it stops people unnecessarily from doing what they want to do.

During his lifetime, Norman Cousins was an excellent role model of health and well-being. Cousins told the true story of his remarkable recovery from a serious disease in his inspiring book, *Anatomy of an Illness*. He was diagnosed with a collagen disease and was told that he had only a 1 in 500 chance for recovery. Instead of giving up and waiting to die, he got busy with his own recovery.

Cousins was aware of the negative impact stress has on the body. He believed that stress had triggered his disease. So, he reasoned, if stress does negative things to the body, why can't the opposite emotions have a positive impact? If stress kills, why can't love, self-confidence, the will to live, faith, and laughter heal? Cousins tested his theory in part by viewing Marx brothers movies and Candid Camera Classics. He found that a ten-minute belly laugh gave him two hours of pain-free sleep. And after each episode of laughter his blood sedimentation rate—the chemical indicator of his disease— dropped. The drop was small, but it held and was cumulative. Cousins laughed himself to a total recovery.

Norman Cousins refused to blindly accept a negative prognosis. If he had chosen acceptance rather than adaptation, he would have resigned himself to progressive paralysis and death. Instead, he chose to look for an answer to his problem. His lack of acceptance led to his eventual recovery.

The opposite of acceptance is denial. And just as there are both healthy and unhealthy forms of acceptance, there are likewise healthy and unhealthy forms of denial. Cousins found a healthy way to deny his prognosis. Sometimes it is difficult to distinguish between a healthy and an unhealthy denial. Parents often ignore a child's vague complaint of a "tummy ache," hoping to discourage the use of illness as an attention-getter or a responsibility-avoider. Obviously, sometimes you should pay attention to a tummy ache. A friend of mine who is a pediatrician missed her son's appendicitis with the "oh-you'll-be-just-fine" approach!

Denial is unhealthy when it leads to unhealthy consequences. Denial of disease can lead to a worsening of the disease if the individual doesn't take medication and follow other healthy behaviors necessary to control it. It's hard to deny health challenges that have obvious outward signs, such as the use of a cane or walker, but many diseases are invisible, causing only internal effects and possibly vague physical symptoms. Hypertension (high blood pressure) is called "the silent killer" because it causes few if any symptoms. Denying it can be deadly. Likewise, a woman who detects a breast lump but does not have it checked is denying its possible threat at great risk to her future well-being.

Diabetes is another insidious killer and crippler, which can be denied for years with little negative consequence. Then, after years of high blood sugars, people can suffer devastating consequences, such as blindness and kidney failure. The irony is that some people feel that by taking care of their disease they are giving in to it and allowing it to take control of their lives. Healthy people realize that by learning how to take care of their disease and then following the required healthy behaviors they are taking control not only of their disease but of their life as well.

Seek a healthy balance between denial and acceptance. Each of us must find our own level of comfort and balance. If you're unsure about the healthiness of your denial, talk it over with a trusted advisor such as your physician.

## Adaptability requires practicality

A practical and realistic attitude about one's disease is the starting point from which to discover healthy adaptations to it.

> I heard of a man whose hand had been seriously burned when he was a child. Because he did not receive the necessary plastic surgery, his hand is now permanently partially closed. Anyone who has tried getting along with just one hand for any length of time knows what a problem that is. But this man handled his challenge with a wonderfully practical approach: "Problems by definition can be solved. My hand is not a problem to me. It is a fact of life. I just do as much as I can with it and do the rest with my other hand."

Try taking this man's approach: think of your disease as he does his partially closed hand. Take practical measures to adapt to the challenge; do not concentrate on the problems. Do as much as you can with your disease, and do the rest with your "other hand," which is everything not affected by your disease.

Dr. William Menninger of the Menninger Foundation and Clinic composed a list he called, "Criteria for Emotional Maturity." The first criterion on the list is: "The ability to deal constructively with reality." That is an excellent definition of adaptability. The entire list appears in the stress management chapter.

Dealing constructively with reality means avoiding the pitfall of "If only. . ." People who fall into this trap spend their whole life saying, "If only things were different, then I would be happy." The thought can take many forms: If only I were married (or single); If only I had a child (or some child-free time to myself); If only I had a new house, a new job, a new wardrobe, a different spouse, a disease-free body. If only (fill in the blank), then my life would be good.

"If only" is not reality. The people who successfully avoid this pitfall are those who make the best of any situation. They successfully adapt their lifestyle to fit their income. They get busy finding things to like about their job, their spouse, and their home. They look beyond the negative to find the positive. They continue to find fulfillment in life even after they get a disease.

> We have to take reality as it comes to us: there is no good jabbering about what it ought to be like or what we should have expected it to be like.
>
> —C.S. Lewis

## Disease is a detour, not a destination

Disease or disability does not have to be a destination or an end point in one's life. Death is surely an end point, but to resign oneself to death because a disease or disability has entered one's life is to deny life itself.

This book addresses living well with health challenges that are chronic in nature, that is, they occur over a long period of time. That generally means an individual who gets a chronic disease lives with it for months or years. The disease is not a destination in itself. Life does not end with the disease, but because it is chronic, the disease becomes part of one's life. Because most diseases present challenges to life and living, they do need to be viewed realistically as detours.

Viewing disease or disability as a detour means that your goal for a fulfilling life remains the same, but the path leading to that goal has been blocked. In order to adapt, you must find an alternate route to reach that goal.

Exploration is essential if you are going to find a way around your roadblock. Explore your disease and learn all that is required for you to live well with it. Explore healthy living in general and, as much as possible, integrate the requirements of your disease with the recommendations of healthy living. Explore yourself. It is essential that you understand your values, needs, and goals.

I have heard many people express the opinion that a benefit they derived from having a disease is the clarity it brings in defining what's *really* important in life. Being confronted by a disease brings people face-to-face with their mortality. Sometimes it is only after this kind of confrontation that people make delightful discoveries like:

- how sweet the spring air smells after a rain
- the exquisite beauty of each unique snowflake
- the priceless melody in a child's laugh
- the profound satisfaction in loving and being loved.

This kind of confrontation can also help people discern what is only superficially important and what is really important in helping them to reach their life's goal. I observed a blind friend of mine as she overcame the obstacle of blindness to reach her life's goal of being a good mother.

She had lost her sight when her daughter was in first grade. Among her greatest struggles with her blindness was the feeling that it diminished her as a mother. This feeling of sadness and loss caused her to closely examine her role as a mother.

She realized she had held the opinion that "a good mother develops her child's curiosity and intelligence through reading." Beginning to view her blindness as a detour, she realized that she could still encourage her daughter's reading without doing the reading herself. My friend and her daughter enjoyed many hours cuddling on the sofa as they listened to cassette tapes of great children's literature.

Sometimes it takes extraordinary determination to adapt to one's challenge. One of my heroes demonstrated this determination in adapting to life with one arm.

Dick is a physician and father of four. He has had only one arm since he was 11 months old, when he stuck his arm into the wringer of his mother's washing machine. Every step along the path of his life required adaptation: learning to tie his shoes, playing baseball, and, of course, the many challenges he met in medical school.

Family support was crucial to Dick's adaptability. His parents insisted that he learn to tie his shoes like the other five year olds. His father spent many hours teaching him how to catch a baseball, quickly get the glove off and throw the ball. Dick lettered in high school baseball.

By the time Dick entered medical school, he truly viewed his challenge as only a detour. During the surgical rotation he tied his surgical mask with one hand and found every other alternative route necessary to take him to the goals he set for himself.

## Learn by observing others

Through appreciation we make the excellence in others our own property.

—Voltaire

Besides receiving inspiration from the stories of brave people who have adapted to their health challenge, you can also learn helpful and practical techniques for adapting to your own challenge.

People with arthritis can find that mobility problems need not make them immobile. By allowing extra time, planning a route that does not present obstacles such as steep stairs, and asking for the support of helpful friends and relatives, the challenge to adapt can be met.

People with digestive disorders can enjoy restaurant eating by finding restaurants that serve appropriate food or are willing to prepare food as the customer requires.

It would be impossible to describe all the adaptations required of individuals with a chronic health challenge. You need to explore and discover ways to adapt to your own challenges, and a good way to start is by observing how others with your disease or disability adapt to their challenges.

To find those individuals, look in your phone book under the disease or disability you have. If there is a local branch of a national organization like the American Cancer Society, Arthritis Foundation, Diabetes Association, Heart Association, or other group, call them. Find out what services they provide. If they hold educational meetings or support groups, attend them. Meet people who are adapting successfully to your health challenge and learn how they do it. If there is no such group in your community, ask at the public library for the address of the national headquarters for your disease. Write and ask them to send information about living with the disease and about the services they provide. Find out what it would take to set up a local branch in your community.

After observing others and reflecting on what you have seen, you will be ready to *apply* what you have learned. Try different techniques, and if they help you, keep at it. Then *evaluate*. If a particular adaptation is not helpful, then keep exploring until you find techniques that do help you adapt successfully.

Nothing in this book is an absolute. Everything must be explored, reflected upon, applied, and evaluated by *you*. That's how to learn to adapt. It is a continuing process because life is ever-changing. The challenges arise. The detours change. Even the goals evolve over time. The only healthy answer is to be able to continually adapt to maintain your well-being and your progress toward your goal of a fulfilling life.

Adaptability provides hope that you will reach your destination. And, at its best, it helps you enjoy the journey.

## Summary

- Adaptability is one of the most helpful assets a person can have, because life's circumstances are always changing. Some people naturally adapt to major changes better than others, but everyone can learn to improve his or her ability to adapt in order to live well with a chronic disease.

- Everyone faces the challenge of physical limitations—it's called aging. Just as aging requires a positive yet realistic approach to living life to its fullest, so does a chronic disease require a positive determination to adapt and do as much as possible with all that one has.

- A highly skilled and committed team of health care providers can be your key to successful adaptation to a chronic illness.

- There is a healthy way of denying disease as well as an unhealthy way. Denial is unhealthy when it leads to a worsening of your disease or detracts from your ability to live well. Denial is healthy when it motivates you to do everything possible to live fully and take control of your disease.

- Successful adapters are busy finding things to like about every part of life. They take a practical approach to doing as much as they can with whatever limitations they have been handed in life.

- Disease is a detour, not a destination.

- Learn from others who have successfully adapted to life with the disease you have by observing them and reflecting on what you have seen. Then apply that information to your life, and, after awhile, evaluate its effectiveness.

## Reflection Questions

1. Make a list of the requirements placed on you by your disease.

Medications:

Therapy:

Diet:

Exercise:

Changes in lifestyle:

Other:

2. Write a description of how you work these requirements into a happy, fulfilling life. This is the first step in adapting!

# CHAPTER 5

# You and Stress: Who's in Control?

The phone never stops ringing at work. There are more orders than you can possibly process. Your manager is pushing you to keep up. You work overtime. As soon as you walk in the door at home, your spouse begins to complain about your being late. You open your mail and learn your parents plan to visit you and stay for three weeks. Your muscles tighten. You're experiencing . . .

## STRESS.

Life is going relatively smoothly for you. You enjoy your work. Your family life is fulfilling. You enjoy leisure activities. Your carefully planned investments are beginning to show the promise of a comfortable retirement. Then you visit your physician for a routine examination. You are told that you have a chronic, incurable disease. The message is clear. It can't be fixed. It might be controllable. It will change the way you live. Your eyes fill with tears as you respond to

## *STRESS.*

This chapter looks at two discrete aspects of stress—that which applies to living with a chronic disease and that which applies to daily living. A disease is a specific stressor and needs specific management techniques. Day-to-day living is more generic but no less a source of stress. Management of daily stress is important not only for your general comfort but also as a preventive measure in managing your existing health problem.

In this chapter, I hope to help you discover the stress created by your health problem and your daily life; explore, choose, and apply techniques to successfully manage that stress; and to help you evaluate the effectiveness of the techniques you choose.

### The physical stress of a disease

Nearly every chronic disease is capable of producing physical signs of stress. These can include, but are not limited to: angina (heart pain), joint pain, discomfort of high or low blood sugar, breathing difficulty, muscle weakness and fatigue, and so on, depending upon the particular ailment.

Your medical team is the best resource for help in addressing the physical signs of stress. They can prescribe medications and treatments and will educate you on how to take the medications and carry out the treatments. They will teach you to watch for early warning signals, avoid things that trigger physical problems, and follow all the recommendations for general good health. The day-to-day and hour-by-hour responsibility for the management of your disease is yours. That responsibility itself can bring on stress.

## The psychological and emotional stress of a disease

Ultimately it is empowering to take on the responsibility for one's life, but there are times in our lives when the very word *responsibility* seems burdensome. We don't want to take responsibility for a disease; we want to be rid of it!

It is normal to feel a sense of loss—the loss of a formerly healthy self. Quite commonly people experiencing this sense of loss go through a grieving process similar to the one Elisabeth Kübler Ross identified in people grieving the death of a loved one. This process can include disbelief, anger, sadness, denial, alternating hopefulness and hopelessness, and finally, acceptance. It is then that we can assume responsibility again and **move forward through our challenge.**

Some people are diagnosed with a chronic disease and see it as their "excuse" to finally take better care of themselves by eating more sensibly, exercising regularly, and managing stress more positively. Other people are diagnosed with a chronic disease and immediately start planning their funeral. One person sees the disease as an opportunity, the other as a disaster. **Stress is not an event. It is our perception of the event.** Of the following five words, which best describes the way you think of your disease?

## Disaster   Burden   Problem   Challenge   Opportunity

Since thoughts can create feelings, explore what feelings you experience when you think of your disease in one of these terms. Thoughts of disaster or burden can promote feelings of depression and hopelessness. If these are your thoughts, then talk with a trusted counselor or a member of your medical team. You won't have the energy to cope if you're stuck in hopelessness.

By talking, you can discover why you view your disease as a disaster or burden. Often this view comes from the fear that a fulfilling life is no longer possible. Through ongoing education and discussion with both medical experts and "real life experts" (the people who live successfully with the same disease), thoughts can change from disaster to problem or challenge as you discover how to adapt. If you can maintain a positive self-image and adapt successfully to the continuous requirements of your disease, then it will not be an overwhelming source of stress to you. **Listen to your thoughts. Talk sense to yourself.** Here is how a woman named Georgia learned to take responsibility for her thoughts and her life.

When Georgia got diabetes, she was both angry and sad. She loved rich desserts and was sad to think she must now give them up. For awhile she was mostly sad as she counted her losses. Then she grew dissatisfied with all the sadness in her life, and, after talking with her medical team and several close friends, she began to practice a technique of choosing different thoughts. Following is a description of how she talks to herself when she begins to feel sad that she cannot eat a rich dessert:

"Oh, how I miss pecan pie! Well, the truth is, I simply can't eat it anymore because I have diabetes. Actually, no one should eat it. It has an enormous number of calories—nearly 800. That's more than half the number of calories I need in a whole day. Those calories, though, are not nutritious, vitamin, mineral, and fiber-filled calories. They are sugary, fatty, empty calories. I am much better off with my new lifestyle of healthy, nutritious eating.

"There are consequences for nearly everything we do. The consequences of eating pecan pie include the risk of gaining weight, having high blood sugars and contributing to the artery-clogging effect of eating saturated fat. A few moments of sweet taste are not worth those risks. Now, instead of sitting here and thinking about pie, what can I do that would be fun? I think I'll call Anne and see if she'd like to walk around the lake. It will be nice to see Anne, to see how the trees are blooming, and a walk will be invigorating and healthy! I am a strong and intelligent person. I have just made a healthy, wise choice."

Dr. George Vaillant, one of the foremost authorities in the United States on adult development, draws this conclusion from his research: "Stress does not kill us so much as ingenious adaptation to stress facilitates our survival." Make an ingenious adaptation to your disease by giving yourself life-enhancing messages to replace the detracting ones. It isn't easy. You will need all the support you can muster. Later chapters will discuss techniques and resources for gaining that support.

If you feel that you are not making progress in managing the stress of your disease, then please, seek counseling. That is a wise step toward well-being, because counselors are excellent teachers of ingenious adaptations to stress. If you are experiencing one or more of the following feelings and situations, you may be depressed and could benefit from professional support.

Feelings of helplessness and hopelessness, feeling trapped.

Sad feelings and crying without knowing why or for very minor reasons.

Feeling confused and unable to make decisions.

Finding it difficult to function in daily routines.

Withdrawal from others, wanting to be left alone.

Dependence on chemicals such as sleeping pills, tranquilizers, or alcohol to keep you going.

Feeling worthless.

Getting caught up in feelings of resentment or self-pity.
                                        —Lutheran Social Services

The diagnosis of a disease can cause a great deal of initial stress. However, stress related to your disease can recur throughout your life. You will never master your disease any more than you will ever master life. Even though you have no control over getting a disease, you can control how much stress it will cause you.

Perceiving your disease as a challenge rather than an insurmountable obstacle will help you cope with it and the stress it causes.

## Disease-related stress throughout life

Because I was a child when I was diagnosed with diabetes, it was my mother who had most of the stress to manage. Because she did that so beautifully, I managed very well. When I got into my teens, I began to assume more of the care-taking responsibility and also to experience more of the stress.

When I was 17, I became eligible for a travel-study program through my high school. But when I reviewed the program's requirements, I read "Diabetics and epileptics need not apply." I was furious! That was SO unfair. Then I was asked by the selection committee to serve as a member of that group in choosing a student for the program. "Why, they've taken a disappointment and turned it into an honor," my mother quickly pointed out to me. I am convinced of that. My new "perception" alleviated my stress.

When I was thinking of getting married I was experiencing stress as I thought of all the terrible things diabetes could do to me and what that would mean for a husband. Before becoming engaged I went to see my physician. I wanted him to give me a definitive answer. I wanted to hear either "Do not get married, because there is always the possibility that you won't do well," or "Go ahead and get married, because I know you are going to do well and live happily ever after."

In a very caring way, my wonderful physician talked sense to me.

He told me that absolutely no one knows what the future will bring. Today's decisions are made without any guarantees about tomorrow. I came to realize that:

*A health challenge does not make life any more uncertain; it simply makes us aware of the uncertainty of life.*

## What is the worst thing that could happen?

A chronic disease does bring with it an awareness of uncertainty. It places expectations we may have had for life in question. My expectations for life included some pretty basic things like working at the job of my choice, getting married, having children, taking occasional vacations. One of the most difficult uncertainties I faced because of my diabetes was my chance to have a child. I was painfully aware that the major complication of a diabetic pregnancy was stillbirth. (Today those risks are greatly diminished because of improved methods of managing diabetes.)

When I was pregnant I could very easily have lived each day in fear of my baby's death. Fear is disabling. I could not enjoy the adventure of pregnancy if I lived in daily fear. So I decided to confront my fear by asking myself these questions: What is the worst thing that can happen? What would I do if it did?

As I thought about these difficult questions, I realized that if I were to lose my baby, I would need another plan for my life. I decided that I would go back to graduate school. I acknowledged to myself that the loss of a baby would be terrible but that we would survive it. Recalling the past experience of my father's death helped me to believe that it is possible to survive tragic loss.

Then I did all that I could do to manage my diabetes and live a healthy life, and faith took care of my lingering anxiety.

Our beautiful son was born, but that did not end the stress that diabetes can provoke.

Because I value motherhood so highly, I experienced some of my most powerful and poignant struggles with diabetes as I perceived it threatening that role. I nursed my baby. While I nursed, my blood sugars would often get low as my body used up calories for milk production.

One night I awakened to John's fiercely hungry cry. As I jumped out of bed, I realized that my blood sugar was low. Because the maternal instinct to tend to my baby was so strong, I seriously considered nursing him first, then eating later. As I walked toward his bedroom, however, I realized that I was very hypoglycemic, so I detoured downstairs for a quick glass of juice. When I got to John's room, I found my husband holding our squalling bit of humanity, trying to comfort him. Dale had figured that I needed to boost my blood sugar, and as he gently rocked John he said to him, "Sometimes Mom has to eat first."

That nearly broke my heart. Moms don't do anything first, or so my culture has taught me. That was a sad moment in my life. However, by the clear light of dawn I was able to talk sense to myself and return some balance to my perception of the situation. I reminded myself that when my blood sugar is low I am vulnerable emotionally and thus would perceive the situation as being far more dire than it actually was. Then I sort of took myself by the shoulders and said, "That's right. Sometimes, in order to be a good mother, you *do* have to eat first, but you're still a good mom." I sincerely felt the issue to be settled, the stress resolved. Again, it is the perception of the event that creates or removes stress.

Your disease must likewise be taken into account as you face every major life event. Your thoughts can take you from anger to understanding, from sadness to a tolerable frustration, and even from doubt to hope.

Successful management of day-to-day stress is important to everyone who wishes to live a healthy, happy life. And successful stress management is even more important for people who have a disease. Unmanaged stress can make an existing disease worse. Unhealthy ways of coping with stress, such as smoking, drinking, and eating, can worsen one's disease. The rest of this chapter will help you define the daily stresses in your life and will discuss ways to control how much stress they cause you.

**The stress of life: dis-ease**

Whether it is family life, work life, social life, or personal life, no one ever reaches a point where they are no longer confronted with challenges. (Think about this: If you suddenly found yourself with no challenges, that in itself would be stressful, because you would need to find some meaningful direction for your life.) Stress produced by life's challenges is not only inevitable, it is essential for fulfillment. A challenge can either be a positive or a negative form of stress, depending on how you perceive it and cope with it. A violin provides an excellent analogy of the importance of stress in one's life. If violin strings have no stress (tension), then the violin can produce no music. But you know what happens when too much stress is applied to the violin's strings: They snap. We need to maintain balance to enjoy the symphony of life! When that balance is lost, we experience "dis-ease," which is psychological, emotional, or spiritual discomfort.

## Know your stress signals

How can you tell when balance is disrupted and the stress in your life has gotten out of hand? What are the signals that alert you? Some common signals include headache, short temper, fatigue, feeling anxious, diarrhea, aching muscles, neck soreness, and jaw pain. You may experience a flare-up of the symptoms of your disease.

Know yourself. People experience stress very differently. Some people always experience headaches, some people never do. For some, the first clue of excessive stress is an increase in a behavior they use to cope with stress. Thus, one person's signal may be an increase in drinking. Another's may be a tendency to snack constantly. Once you become aware of your stress signal, figure out what is causing the stress.

## What drains your battery? What energizes it?

To assess the sources of stress in your life, think of your *life force* as a battery. On a daily basis, the various events of life drain that battery but they also can energize it. On a regular basis, do the following activity:

Place a minus sign at the top left of a sheet of paper and a plus sign at the top right. Under the minus sign list all of the current **drains** in your life. Energy drains come in many forms: deadlines to meet, too much work, unsatisfactory relationships, loss of a job or a loved one—any of the many "hassles" of daily living. Under the plus sign list all the current **energizers** in your life. Energizers also come in many forms: stimulating, fulfilling work, satisfying relationships, a vacation, a good book or movie, lively music, a great joke.

Now look at these two lists. Do they balance each other? (You may want to assign numbers to each item, indicating its relative value.) As you analyze the lists, try to determine whether you are receiving enough energy from life to offset the drains and provide you with the energy you need to live a fulfilling life. The following list of possible drains and energizers are part of the battery exercise that I have conducted all over the United States, Canada, and Australia with a wide variety of groups: people with chronic disease, health professionals, and business people.

| DRAINS | ENERGIZERS |
|---|---|
| − | + |
| building a house | kids |
| entertaining | exercise |
| cynical attitudes | relationship |
| indecision | a raise |
| unemployed spouse | fellowship |
| deadlines | learning |
| threat of layoff | good friend |
| procrastination | music |
| being a perfectionist | solitude |
| parenting | prayer |
| change | recognition |
| studying | nature |
| single marital status | unscheduled time |
| death of a loved one | sunny weather |
| finances | undisturbed bath time |
| lack of support | laughter |
| traffic | unallocated money |
| pessimistic people | celebrations |
| housework | random acts of kindness |
| politics | promotions |
| family conflict | vacations |
| elderly parent | birth of a child |
| | good novel |
| | triplet grandchildren |
| | sleep |
| | pets |
| | thoughts of a free world |

There are a number of things you can learn from doing this exercise. Sometimes the same person or event can be both an energizer and a drain. Holidays are enjoyable *and* they're a lot of work. Family members whom we love dearly can be a drain due to illness or other trials. If we allow ourselves to feel guilty for viewing loved ones as drains, then we experience that additional drain brought on by guilt. Use this activity as an awareness-raising exercise that sets the stage for some goal setting that can restore balance.

Do the battery exercise whenever you have a vague sense of being anxious or stressed. It can help you to figure out why. Then you can choose what to do about it. To use the battery exercise to *prevent* stress from getting the upper hand, do it regularly—the first of every month, every Sunday evening, whatever works best for you. You may find it helpful to have your calendar with you. As you draw up your list, look not only at the current month but also at the month before and after. You may discover some lingering stress from the previous month (a letter you intended to write and didn't) as well as some stress caused by something coming up the following month.

Another lesson many learn from this exercise is that although they can think of plenty of energizers, they don't give them to themselves. It does you no good to simply list things that give you energy unless you are actively incorporating them into your life. And they also learn that drains don't have to be huge to be bothersome. Some stress management experts believe that chronic small irritations are ultimately more stressful and take a greater toll than occasional major stress. So list everything, and keep adding energizers until they *clearly* outweigh your drains.

## Reduce the drains in your life

Look over the list of drains in your life. Decide which ones are problems that can be solved and then put them through the problem-solving process covered in chapter 6. There are times when you may experience what is called "episodic" stress, when for a brief time there is an unavoidable stress (tax time, house guests). The knowledge that the stress will end helps you to cope with the temporary discomfort.

Obviously, there are drains in everyone's life over which we have little or no control—the tragic news of a loved one's death, the loss of a job, the local, national, and world crises covered daily in the news. Though we cannot always control the drains and stresses, we can control how much of an impact they will have on our lives. One way we diminish the impact of drains is by increasing the energizers. We don't always control the drains; we do control the energizers because we can choose to incorporate them into our lives.

## Increase your energizers

The basic philosophy behind increasing energizers is that they serve as a buffer against all the stressors and drains. *Energizers help you to prevent the harmful effects of stress.* The fuller your cup, the more easily you can withstand a little drain now and then. Use the following energizers to both prevent and treat stress in your life:

## Self-talk

Thoughts create feelings. To relieve stressful feelings, explore new thoughts to alter your perceptions. (The practice of changing negative to positive thoughts and feelings is discussed, you will recall, in chapter 2.) When my husband was working hard to get his new business going, he came home one day looking extremely tired. He said to me, "I'll bet the phone rang 200 times today!" Then, before I could respond, he grinned and said, "Business is good!"

One of my favorite perspectives on the subject of the benefits of work-related stress is that of the Reverend John Wesley Ford:

> Be thankful for the troubles of your job. They provide about half your income, because if it were not for the things that go wrong, the difficult people you have to deal with, and the problems and unpleasantness of your working day, someone could be found to handle your job for half of what you are being paid.

> It takes intelligence, resourcefulness, patience, tact, and courage to meet the troubles of any job. That is why you hold your present job. If all of us would start to look for more troubles and learn to handle them cheerfully and with good judgment as opportunities rather than irritation, we would find ourselves getting ahead at a surprising rate, for it is a fact that there are plenty of big jobs waiting for those who aren't afraid of the troubles connected with them.

## Exercise

Choose a physical activity suitable to your specific needs and one you enjoy. That adds *fun*, which is another great stress reducer! For those who can, a good, brisk, arm-swinging walk is one of the best exercises. Vigorous exercise should be cleared with your doctor. (Exercise should reduce stress, not create it!) Increase your enjoyment by inviting a friend to join you. You'll be more likely to exercise regularly, and you'll also be promoting your friend's health.

## Laughter

Make your own list of the sources of laughter in your life, such as funny movies, friends, books, games, and events. Remember, Socrates' philosopher friend Phaedrus said, "The mind ought sometimes to be amused, that it may the better return to thought, and to itself." And Proverbs says, "A merry heart doeth like good medicine, but a broken spirit drieth the bones" (17:22).

## Vacation

Take a real vacation—completely cut off from your daily routine—on a regular basis. Everyone needs to renew, recharge, and relax.

## Music

Music has been a source of enjoyment for centuries. The Greeks believed music brought harmony within the body, mind, and soul, and between people. Apollo was the god of music and medicine. Today, music therapists use music to increase well-being in people with special needs. Much of the current work is done at either end of the age spectrum: the elderly and the newborn. Music is used to help Alzheimer's patients gain access to their memories. It is used in newborn nurseries to calm babies.

For those of us on the continuum between the newly born and elderly, we can allow our intuition to guide us toward music that will soothe when we need soothing and ignite when we need inspiration. During one particularly extended period of stress in my life, I kept Judy Collins' "Amazing Grace" on the turntable of my stereo. Almost daily I sat with my eyes closed listening to her lovely a cappella voice singing the promise of amazing grace. And I've learned I'm not the only person who sings along to music on the radio and occasionally performs by lipsync. So, besides relaxation and inspiration, music can provide a fun escape.

## Relaxation Techniques

Find a quiet place where you are comfortable and can be undisturbed for 20 minutes. Sit awhile with your eyes closed. Get a picture in your mind of a huge gunny sack and, one by one, drop all of your worries and burdens into it. Begin a progressive muscle relaxation exercise, starting with your scalp and facial muscles. Alternately tighten each muscle group and then relax it. Go to the next muscle group and continue this technique of flexing for several seconds, then releasing and relaxing the muscles, group by group, until you reach your toes.

You may want to do progressive relaxation to relaxing music of your choice. Some people record their own voice giving them instructions to tighten and relax the specific muscle groups.

For a quick relaxer, try deep breathing. Slowly take in a deep breath through your nose—as much air as you possibly can. Hold it to the count of six, then slowly let all the air out through your mouth. When I do this, I tell myself on the inhale that I am breathing in energy. On the exhale, I tell myself that I am expelling all my stress. It works!

## Visualization

Once you are in a relaxed state, you are ready to experience further relaxation through visualization, which was discussed in chapter 3 as a motivational tool. It is also a powerful stress reducer. To do this, remember a time and place where you felt relaxed and happy. Close your eyes. "See" yourself relaxed and happy at your chosen location. Now, remember it with all your senses. What do you see, hear, feel, smell, taste? Here's an example of my favorite visualization:

> I see myself sitting next to a fire on a beach. I am smiling and I look peaceful. I hear the crackling of the wood as it burns. I also hear the waves lapping on the shore. I feel the heat from the fire. I also feel the cool, silky sand as I run my toes and fingers through it. I smell the smoke of the fire and the distinct, but pleasant smell of the river. I am at peace. I am relaxed.

Have mental pictures that are very soothing and appealing. Visit them often, as if you were taking a brief vacation. Keep pictures of your favorite place on your desk or countertop to remind you to take that mini-vacation.

> Location for relaxation:
> Choice of background music:
> Favorite visualization:
>
> I see . . .
>
> I hear . . .
>
> I smell . . .
>
> I feel . . .
>
> I taste . . .
>
> I am relaxed.

Besides visualizing, keep dreaming. Dreaming about your lifetime goals and desires is also important in day-to-day coping. Dreams lift us above our troubles and give us hope. As Langston Hughes expresses it:

> Hold fast to dreams
> For if Dreams die
> Life is a broken-winged bird
> That cannot fly.
>
> Hold fast to dreams
> For when dreams go
> Life is a barren field
> Frozen with snow.

## Meditation

Meditation is a spiritual activity that may have no connection to religion. Words like "unseen" and "innermost" are frequently associated with the spiritual. During meditation, people spend time, usually alone and in a quiet place, seeking wisdom, insight, peace, and other spiritual outcomes. Meditation is deep reflection in which we listen to our inner voice.

## Prayer

Prayer is usually connected to a religious belief. It is communication or connection with God. People report that through prayer, they let go of whatever problems they have, believing that a loving, wise, powerful, and gracious God will give them the help they need. Fellowship is another aspect of religion that people say is important. Coming together to worship with people of a like faith is frequently included in descriptions of how people manage stress.

Senator Sam J. Ervin, Jr., offered this interesting thought regarding religion and stress:

> Religious faith is not a storm cellar to which men and women can flee for refuge from the storms of life. It is, instead, an inner spiritual strength that enables them to face those storms with hope and serenity. Religious faith has the miraculous power to lift ordinary human beings to greatness in seasons of stress. Religious faith is to be found in the promises of God.

The following is a translation of a Japanese variation of the 23rd Psalm:

> The Lord is my pace-setter, I shall not rush.
> He makes me stop and rest for quiet intervals;
> He provides me with images of stillness
> which restore my serenity.
> He leads me in the ways of efficiency through
> calmness of mind,
> And His guidance is my peace.
> Even though I have a great many things
> to accomplish each day,
> I will not fret, for His presence is here.
> His timelessness, His all-importance, will keep me in balance.

He prepares refreshment and renewal in the midst of my
activity
By anointing my mind with His oils of tranquility.
My cup of joyous energy overflows.
Surely harmony and effectiveness shall be the fruit of my
hours,
For I shall walk in the pace of my Lord
and dwell in His house forever.

—Toki Miyashina

(Reproduced by kind permission of The Saint Andrew Press, Edinburgh,
Scotland.)

## Support network

Select a friend who has experienced the type of stress you are
experiencing—preferably one who has successfully overcome it.
Talk about it. Express your feelings. Telling a trusted friend
what's bothering you helps to clarify your thoughts. And you
may find a resolution for the stress as you listen to yourself. If no
one in your support system seems to understand you, do not
hesitate to get professional counseling.

Be part of someone else's support network. Hans Selye, physician and noted stress management expert, considered this to be
one of the most important ways to manage stress. He called it
"altruistic egotism." When we help others, we help ourselves.
Many charitable organizations and agencies need your help.
Perhaps the most gratifying giving is that which is done in person.
Find someone you can visit, cheer up, or help in any way.

One of our son's friends broke his leg in a hockey game. He had to be in traction in the hospital for more than two weeks. It was a tough time for an 11-year-old boy and his family. Instinctively, we reached out to this family, and as we did, we felt our own continued healing. This is part of the letter I wrote our young friend when he left the hospital:

> You will never be the same person because of your broken leg. You are a better, stronger, wiser person. You may not be aware of that yet. But, someday you will hear of a little boy who has broken his leg (playing hockey, skiing, or in a car accident) and is hospitalized in traction. Your heart will tell you what you have to do. It is then that you will understand the special gift you have to help another person to heal. You will also discover that in helping someone else you have helped yourself toward greater healing and continued growth. As is true of love, the more you give, the more you receive.

I like the term "wounded healer." A special healing touch belongs only to those who have been wounded.

## Prevention

(It's still worth a pound of cure any day!)

Set priorities for yourself. Make a list of all the tasks you perform, and then read through and think about each item. Star those that are essential (going to work, grocery shopping, paying bills, child care, housework, etc.). Check those that are important to you (weekly bowling, singing in a group, attending your child's school events, seeing friends, etc.). Consider the remaining items to be unimportant. Cut them out of your life. Be very careful before you say "yes" to any more responsibilities. Say "no" to things that will overload your stress budget. If you have a tendency to completely fill your calendar, block some time out for relaxation. Remind yourself that relaxation is not an extravagance, but rather an essential part of life.

Learn to manage your time well. An excellent, highly readable guide to both priority setting and time management is the book *How to Get Control of Your Time and Your Life*, by Alan Lakein. When time is not well managed, stress is too often the result. However, when people manage time well, they frequently experience the fulfilling sense of being in control of their lives.

## Evaluation

Evaluate the effectiveness of your coping methods. Do you feel better? If you feel better, that is, less stressed, then perhaps you have dealt successfully with your stress. However, feeling better cannot be the only measure of successful stress management. Some people say they feel better after getting drunk or abusing their spouse. It is important that your stress management techniques yield positive and healthy benefits for you and those close to you. The goal is to have an overall positive impact on your well-being.

## Knowledge

Continue on your own to seek more information on stress and its successful management. I have especially enjoyed the insights of Dr. Vaillant, whom I mentioned earlier in the chapter. He recommends the following ways of coping with change and stress: altruism (giving of yourself to help others), sublimation (directing your energy into hobbies and other worthwhile pursuits), and humor.

In your knowledge gathering, seek to understand yourself better. Dr. Alan Marlatt of Washington University encourages self-awareness in his work on the psychology of relapse (restarting a negative behavior). His recommendations include:

1. Know your high-risk situations, those which most commonly cause you to feel stressed.
2. Plan for high-risk situations by deciding ahead of time what stress management methods you will use. See *yourself in the high-risk setting, successfully using your chosen positive behavior to manage the stress it causes.*
3. See your progress on a continuum. If you slip occasionally, realize that it was only a temporary lapse and not a total relapse. People fail when they view their challenge as an all or nothing, win or lose process. Everyone "slips" from time to time. Forgive yourself. Then keep moving forward.

Read and reflect on the following criteria of emotional maturity that were established by William C. Menninger, M.D., of the well-known Menninger Clinic.

Emotional maturity is:

• the ability to deal constructively with reality
• the capacity to adapt to change
• a relative freedom from symptoms that are produced by tensions and anxieties

- the capacity to find more satisfaction in giving than in receiving
- the capacity to relate to other people in a consistent manner with mutual satisfaction and helpfulness
- the capacity to sublimate, that is, to direct one's instinctive hostile energy into creative and constructive outlets
- the capacity to love.

Keep learning, exploring the world around you and within you.

## A tool box for stress

View all of the suggestions in this chapter as tools. You now have a whole box full of tools for stress management. Some will be useful in specific situations but not all the time. You choose which tools will suit your unique needs at different times. A hammer can't do what a saw can do.

Remember that as you choose your stress management tools, if one doesn't work, try another. But remember, just as a hammer and saw cannot make furniture by themselves, neither can these stress management tools benefit you unless you *use them*. Perhaps the most important advice comes from the Ohio Mental Health Association: GUTS, or "Get Underway. Try Something!"

And here's a great bit of advice for avoiding undue stress:

> We must try to take
> life moment by
> moment. The actual
> present is usually pretty
> tolerable, I think, if
> only we refrain
> from adding to its
> burden that of the
> past and the
> future. How
> right our Lord
> is about
> sufficient to the day.

—C.S. Lewis
*Letter to an American Lady*

## Summary

- Stress is an inevitable part of everyone's life. Management of daily stress is important as a preventive measure in managing any health problem.

- Having a disease adds stress to life and requires specific management techniques.

- Stress is not an event. It is our perception of the event.

- If you are not making progress in managing the stress of your disease, seek professional counseling.

- Stress is like a violin: If violin strings have no stress (tension) then the violin can provide no music. But if too much stress is applied to the strings, they snap.

- Know your stress signals—the feelings or behaviors that let you know stress is taking its toll on your well-being.

- Assess the sources of stress in your life by listing those things that drain and energize you. Keep adding energizers until they clearly outweight the drains.

- Try various techniques for coping with stress, remembering that successful stress management requires preventive techniques as well as techniques to lessen the damage from temporary, major sources of stress. Build a tool box full of stress management techniques, and become a master craftsperson with your tools.

## Reflection Questions

1. Identify your high-risk situations.

2. Define the stress management methods you will use to deal with these situations in the future. (Options can be found on pages 106-117.)

3. List the drains and energizers in your life.

After looking at your drains and energizers, decide if your life is out of balance. Describe the action(s) you can take to get your life back in balance.

CHAPTER 6

# Problems
# Are Only
# Detours

You're all set to go on vacation. You plan to drive across the country to visit dear friends. You're really excited! You've traced the route on your map; you're all packed and ready to go. However, shortly after starting out you discover the highway you selected is blocked off because of road repair. Your goal may be Washington state, but roadblocks present a problem in getting there.

Have you encountered "roadblocks" in your life that present problems in reaching your goals? In the first chapter, we explored goal setting. Goals look so easy on paper, but when you leave the abstract realm of paper doodling and apply your plan to concrete life, you often find problems. Sometimes detour signs clearly reroute you so you can continue on your way. Often, however, *you* have to figure it out.

*That's problem solving.*

The classic definition of a problem is "a question raised for solution." I believe that detours fit into that definition because they raise questions like, "Where do I go now? How do I get there?" And these questions lead to solutions, that is, a new route to reach the destination—the goal.

Problems confront everyone, everyday. Some seem fairly simple: getting to work when your car has broken down. Others seem quite complex: making lifestyle changes to accommodate health challenges while still pursuing an enjoyable life. But, whether simple or complex, the process of finding a solution is essentially the same. This chapter will explore the philosophy and practice of problem solving.

## Keep your goal in mind

Reflect for a moment on your goal and on the barriers you encountered in pursuing your goals. The more important your goal is, the harder you'll work at solving any problem that gets in the way. You're likely to work harder, for example, to reach a vacation destination than you would to get to a shopping center. Ask yourself these questions:

*Is reaching this goal important?  Why?*

Knowing why this goal is important to you will reinforce your commitment to solving the problems that get in your way. And, by writing out WHY THIS GOAL IS IMPORTANT, you will strengthen your commitment further.

## Desire, determination, and perseverance

The people who are most likely to find solutions to problems are those who have a strong *desire* to do so. The person who does not have much desire to go to work may view a sick child or broken car as a good excuse to stay home. I've heard stories of paralyzed persons who have become proficient at using a computer because their great desire to go to school or get a job has helped them overcome seemingly insurmountable physical obstacles. If there is a solution to a particular problem, it will be found by the person who desires to find it, the person with an "I can" attitude.

Here is a story that shows the contrast between a problem keeper and a solution finder:

I taught summer school once when I was an English teacher. The basic problem with all the students in that program was that they were reluctant to participate. So, as one of our culminating activities, we planned a three-day canoe trip. For the canoe trip to work, everyone would have to do his or her share of cooking, cleaning up, wood gathering, paddling, and so on.

After weeks of planning we met early one morning to board the bus that would take us to the river. One of the students handed me a note from his father. "Please excuse Jim from the canoe trip. He cannot go because he has diabetes." I was shocked that he felt he couldn't go on the canoe trip. "Jim," I said, "I have diabetes and I'm going!" Jim looked astonished. "Well," he sputtered, "what are you going to do with your insulin and syringes? If the

canoe tips over they'll sink to the bottom of the river!"
"They're in a plastic, air-tight container, Jim. If the canoe
tips, they'll float."

I really wanted to go on that canoe trip. My desire led me
to figure out exactly how to do that. Jim did not want to go,
so he used his diabetes as an excuse to get out of any
school-related activity.

Do some careful self-examination of your desires. Which gives
you greater payoffs, keeping your problems or finding a solution? To nurture your desire to find a solution, keep reminding
yourself of all the positive values you hold. It was love of family
that fueled my friend Molly's desire to find a solution to her
problem. Her renal dialysis fell on Christmas Eve day. Instead
of giving up on the idea of entertaining her family that same day,
she negotiated with the hospital and changed her dialysis to
December 23.

Along with desire, the philosophy of problem solving requires
determination and perseverance. Determination is the strength
and energy you put into your effort, while perseverance is the
duration of the effort. Determination becomes very real to me
when I watch my nephew Eric take five minutes to tie his shoe.
Cerebral palsy makes the otherwise simple task a great challenge
for him. He has the class of determination about which Sir
Winston Churchill spoke when he said, "Never give up. Never,
never." And perseverance adds her message: "Try again, and if
that doesn't work, try again and again and again."

> Perseverance is not a long race;
> it is many short races one after another.
> —Walter Elliot

No one has the strength to always find solutions without help. In upcoming chapters we will examine support, the external and internal strengths that make desire, determination, and perseverance possible. With these important allies you can turn your attention to the practical approach to finding solutions.

## Define your problem

> A problem well-stated is a problem half-solved.
> —Charles F. Kettering

In defining your problem, state it both accurately and specifically. If you state that your problem is your disease, you have not been specific enough. What is it about your disease that is a problem to you? Fear for the future? Frustration over the limitations it has imposed on your present life? Mobility, for example, is not specific enough. A more helpful description of this limitation would be: I can't walk as fast as I want to; stairs are impossibly painful for me; or I'm embarrassed when people stare at me in public because I walk "funny." Take time to specifically and accurately describe your problem.

Another example of too vague a definition is defining the problem as "diabetes" after experiencing an embarrassing insulin reaction in the middle of a social event. By really looking at the situation objectively and honestly, a person would see that the real problem was a lack of preparedness. The reaction could have been avoided if meals and snacks had been eaten on time, exercise had been figured into the day's eating and insulin schedule, and the person had carried something with which to treat the early signs of a reaction. This list of ways in which the reaction could have been avoided is an example of the second step in solution finding.

## List all the things you can do about it

List all the things you can think of that might help solve your problem. If the problem is health-related, you may need assistance from your medical team. But you may have enough knowledge to solve it yourself. People with lupus, multiple sclerosis, arthritis, and other diseases can experience a flare-up of their symptoms if their life becomes too busy or stressful. If making changes in their daily living doesn't reduce the flare-up, the medical team should be consulted.

The same is true for emotional or psychological problems. Sometimes you can solve them by giving yourself a pep talk or changing negative thoughts into positive ones. Other times you may need to turn to a professional counselor for help. Be sure to list all of your options. If one does not help, you need backups to try until you find the right one.

In brainstorming, it is important not to limit yourself. List as many ideas as you can possibly think of. From that kind of a list you will not only find "a" solution, but many solutions. Throughout life we are confronted with the same problems. To keep solving them we need plenty of reinforcements: solutions backing up solutions.

Since healthy eating is an important goal for everyone, let us use that challenge as an example in brainstorming solutions. The specific challenges to eating nutritiously are commonly overeating and making poor food choices. Following is the beginning of some brainstorming:

—In a restaurant, order smaller portions.

—At home, serve plates instead of "family style."

—Eat only what you should, then clear your plate.

—Eat only what you should, then heavily salt what is left on your plate.

—Concentrate on the atmosphere of a restaurant, including decor, music, and conversation.

—At home, get involved with family conversation and slow down your eating.

—At a restaurant, request that the meat portion be halved before it's brought to you with one half placed immediately into a doggie bag.

—Whenever possible, choose dining companions with a similar interest in healthful, sensible eating.

—Select restaurants carefully, avoiding the "all you can eat for one price" variety.

—At home, make only as much as you and your family need, so that there are no "seconds."

—If a recipe makes more than your family needs, put the leftovers into the refrigerator or freezer before you even sit down to eat.

—Immediately after eating, brush your teeth so as to remove the taste of food from your mouth.

—Plan an activity to begin shortly after the meal so that your thoughts will naturally move to that activity and not dwell on food.

—Do not buy junk food or allow it in your home.

—When bored, clean a closet, call a friend, go for a walk; do anything except eat.

—When stressed, look at your list of positive coping choices: use them, not food.

If you find it difficult to brainstorm alone, then do it with a friend, a support group, a member of your medical team or anyone with a similar interest.

## Take action and evaluate

Now that you have a list of numerous options, start trying them. Evaluate as you do this. Is the problem getting solved? If so, you have successfully carried out the process. If not, try another of your options. If other options don't help, perhaps your problem may not have been well defined. Try to be more specific. Upon reflection you may decide that the biggest challenge to healthy eating is your weekend lifestyle. The friends with whom you socialize may serve high fat, salt, and calorie meals. This additional, specific information will help you to think of options that are more liable to solve the problem, like:

   —educate your friends about your eating requirements
   —ask for their support
   —offer to bring a low-fat casserole and fruit plate
   —create and suggest attractive and healthful menus

If you do not find an effective solution, go to your support system (those mentioned in the paragraph above) for assistance before you become discouraged. Here is an illustration of how this process works:

**Problem:** "All I think about is my heart. I'm afraid to do things. I'm afraid that at any moment I will have another heart attack. I am consumed by my health and feel my life is out of balance.

**Options:**
— I will replace my fearful thoughts with positive ones. But, frankly, no matter how many positive thoughts I give myself, that nagging fear is always there and returns day after day. I'll go to another option.
— I will get busy with my hobbies to avoid obsessing about my health. Even though I truly enjoy my hobby of woodworking, I could do it with my eyes closed. Unfortunately, it just doesn't distract me enough to overcome my anxiety.
— I will visit my doctor and openly discuss my concerns. She once gave me some helpful information about cardiac rehabilitation, which relieved some of my fears. Then, she recommended that I visit a counselor. I did and it helped me regain a healthy perspective. My sense of well-being was definitely improved.

Solving this problem was fairly simple, but it required a purposeful approach on the part of the individual. The person defined the problem, described three possible options, and then tried each to find which worked. Let's look at how the same process can work in a more complex example:

**Problem:** "I'm worried. I've lost my job and I'm afraid that I won't find another. My worrying is causing me so much stress that my diabetes is often out of control. On top of that I'm coping with my stress by eating more than I should, adding to my diabetes control problems. I just can't see my way out of this!"

This person is so overwhelmed by the complexity of his problems that there is real danger he may not even be able to list possible solutions, much less act on them. When a problem gets as complex as this one, you must break it down into components. In *How to Get Control of Your Time and Your Life*, Alan Lakein recommends the "Swiss cheese" approach to problem solving. He advises that you break a problem down into smaller parts and then begin to work on one small part at a time. In this way you gradually make enough "holes" in the larger problem to make it fall apart, and it is resolved. So, taking that approach, our friend breaks his problem down like this:

**Problem**: "My basic problem is worry. Specifically, I'm worried about four things:

—about finding a job
—that family and friends will think of me as a loser if I don't get another job real soon
—about the effect this stress is having on my diabetes
—my frustration that I'm coping so poorly. I know better. I just can't seem to get my life together!

**Options for worrying about finding a job**: I will talk sense to myself. Lots of people lose a job and then not only find a new one but one they like even better. I really don't need to worry about finances yet. My wife has an excellent job, and her income can sustain us until I get a position. I'll apply for a teaching job at all the schools close to us. I'll also look outside the teaching profession, because my skills can be applied elsewhere. To bolster my self-confidence for the job hunt, I'll attend community college seminars on resume writing and interviewing.

**Option for worrying about what friends and family will think**: I will again talk sense to myself. My family and friends are well aware of the general trend of declining enrollments in schools. It was my lack of seniority and not a lack of competence that caused me to be laid off. They know that. I will ask for their support. If they were in my shoes they'd want my support.

**Option for worrying about the effects of stress on my diabetes:** I will talk with my doctor and get advice on how to deal with these flare-ups and how to manage my stress more positively.

**Options for my frustration at coping poorly:** I'll get together with Dave and talk about how I feel. He has a unique way of always seeing the positive side of things, and he went through a job change just last year. Also, I'll attend the support group at the diabetes association. Those people always inspire me to believe in my ability to cope well.

I will set a goal of spending at least two hours each day calling around and checking out leads on jobs. And as a reward, I'll visit a museum or go to an afternoon movie each week; this is the time for me to do all those things I daydreamed about during those long afternoons at work. I will forgive myself for past weaknesses at coping. I will give myself positive messages.

### I can cope

As this person moved toward the solution phase of this process an interesting thing had already happened: he was worrying less. Just laying out his problem in small parts and planning options for solving each helped make it all manageable. He began to feel more in control of the situation. He then realized that his stress had immobilized him. Because he was feeling less overwhelmed, he was able to get moving on some of those solutions. Using the "Swiss cheese" approach, he acted on one option after another and solved his problems one by one. Now his worry has all but disappeared.

Sure, there have been setbacks, especially the time he ran into some old pals from college who were having a business lunch to discuss a shared venture between their two companies. Hearing them talk so enthusiastically about their careers and then having to explain that he was out of work was *so* hard. He almost collapsed into self-pity. He cried a little and laughed a little, and then picked himself up and swore that one year from that day he would have lunch at the same restaurant as a happily employed, healthy person.

All the energy he had put into worrying he now puts into finding a new job and balancing his life. And not only is he feeling much better inside, he is a self-confident person on the outside—a fact that he projects strongly in his job interviews.

## Be logical instead of emotional

An important part of effective problem solving is the ability to be logical. Obviously, problems can cause an emotional response in anyone. Deal with the emotion until you can view your problem from a logical rather than emotional perspective. One of the most amazing examples of getting quickly into a logical perspective was when a friend of mine knew moments before he was rear-ended that the accident was about to occur and supported his neck on the back of his car seat. There was no way Steve could have prevented the accident from happening, but his cool, logical problem solving prevented him from receiving serious whiplash.

## Quality of life

The broad, overall issue here is to achieve and maintain a quality of life that takes into account both the demands of your disease and the dreams you have for your life. Whenever a problem arises and threatens your quality of life, put it through the problem solving process: Define your problem, break it down if it seems complex, list your options, take action, and evaluate. To ignite your spirit of determination, remember this thought of Harriet Beecher Stowe:

> When you get into a tight place and it seems that you can't hold on for a minute longer, never give up; for that's just the place and time that the tide will turn.

## Solving the problems of a chronic disease

Some examples of persons with chronic diseases finding solutions to problems may help you make a realistic assessment of your problem:

## Bob Walters

Bob Walters visited his doctor for a routine, quarterly diabetes check-up. The blood test indicated that Bob's diabetes had been poorly controlled. Bob's doctor asked him, "How have things been going for you? Are you aware of any problem that would explain your diabetes being out of control?"

**Defining the Problem**: Bob defined his problem this way: "Diabetes places such heavy demands on our lifestyle that I'm afraid my wife just isn't able to do all the necessary meal preparation." The doctor asked Bob to bring his wife to the next appointment.

As the doctor spoke with Bob and his wife, she sensed a tremendous amount of friction in their relationship. Not only did they speak abruptly to each other, they argued openly about their eating habits. Mrs. Walters insisted that she provided the meals she had been taught to prepare for Bob. She accused Bob of uncontrolled snacking. It was quite apparent to the doctor that diabetes was a problem secondary to their marital problems.

**Finding Options**: The doctor recommended counseling for the Walters.

**Taking Action**: They agreed, and as they progressed through counseling and rehabilitated their relationship, Bob's diabetes management improved.

With the next problem he encountered, Bob was able to analyze the situation himself.

**Defining the Problem**: He realized that stress at work was his real problem. He saw that he was coping with stress by eating, causing his diabetes to go out of control and causing him to gain weight, which was making him lose self-esteem.

**Finding Options**: Bob learned new, more positive coping methods.

**Taking Action**: Realizing how right they were for him, he found the motivation and support to use them.

**Evaluating**: Then he noticed three outcomes of his new behavior: he was controlling his diabetes well, he had achieved a healthy weight, and he felt better about himself as a person.

## Marie Landini

Marie Landini has arthritis. It is important that she do daily stretching exercises to retain mobility in her joints. Her doctor told her that the exercises would be painful at first but that it was absolutely necessary to go through a full range of motion daily. Marie not only failed to make progress in mobility, she actually lost mobility. When her doctor noted this, he asked Marie if she was faithfully doing her exercises.

**Defining the Problem**: Marie reported that it was sometimes so painful that she stopped. The doctor then asked her to demonstrate how she did the exercises. He observed that Marie arched her back and did many adaptive movements with her body, making the exercises almost worthless. They discovered two problems: the pain was causing her to quit too soon, and her technique of exercising was incorrect.

**Finding Options**: The doctor referred Marie to her physical therapist, who helped Marie practice her exercise technique. The therapist also gave her a videotape to take home to use as an instructional aid while she did her exercises, and he recommended she place a full length mirror next to the television so she could compare her technique to that of the instructor.

**Taking Action**: Seeing it done right helped Marie make sure her technique was correct. The videotape also helped distract Marie from the pain. She was able to hold her stretches longer than when she exercised alone.

**Evaluating**: This helped her discover that when she was not able to watch the videotape she could do other things to distract herself, such as reading, watching television, or listening to music while she exercised.

## Dan Hankinson

Dan Hankinson had a heart attack at the age of 47. When he left the hospital, he received instructions on how he should eat, exercise, and manage stress. In a follow-up visit to his doctor, Dan was still very much overweight, his cholesterol level was not declining, and he seemed depressed.

**Defining the Problem**: When Dan's physician asked him how he was doing, Dan said, "I don't know what my problem is. I understand very well what to do and why I need to do it, but I just can't seem to get myself going." After further discussion with his doctor, Dan saw his problem as a lack of conviction about the importance of a wellness lifestyle.

**Finding Options**: Dan's doctor made two recommendations: either join a support group of heart patients or take a wellness seminar offered by the clinic, since virtually all the lifestyle recommendations of the wellness program would help Dan. His doctor felt that the wellness program could reinforce not only the valuable information of a healthy lifestyle, but also the important philosophy that Dan's new lifestyle be one of good health and good sense. Dan's doctor also recommended that he meet another of his patients who was close to Dan's age and had also had a heart attack but was doing well making lifestyle changes and feeling the benefits of increased well-being.

**Taking Action**: Dan's visit with the other patient helped him learn some practical information on overcoming his obstacles and made him better able to define his own problem. He realized when he went out for lunch with his coworkers he was eating poorly. He blamed this on the type of restaurants they usually went to and the fact everyone else ordered high-fat selections and he found it difficult to do differently.

**Finding more options**: Dan gained reinforcement for a healthy lifestyle from the wellness program. And his newfound friend shared some practical suggestions with Dan, such as "Be the first to order, maybe they'll follow the leader and order healthier meals. Suggest another restaurant with healthier selections; tell your coworkers about your need for nutritious meals, be more assertive."

**Evaluating**: To Dan's pleasant surprise, several people he worked with were interested in good health and joined him in ordering a turkey sandwich on whole wheat bread for lunch. An even more pleasant surprise was to feel his depression lift and be replaced by a new enthusiasm for life. And, on his next check-up, his doctor congratulated him on the health improvements he was making.

## Karen Moore

Karen Moore, a teacher, was diagnosed with liver cancer. For months she felt ill as she underwent vigorous therapy. She had to take a leave of absence from teaching. She became very depressed but sensed that her depression was not associated with the fear of dying. Karen's strong religious faith helped her regard death as a new beginning, rather than the end of life. This strong conviction left her confused about her depression. She sought the source of her problem by speaking with her pastor.

**Defining the Problem**: In talking with her pastor, Karen came to realize that her depression was linked to her frustration at not being able to fulfill her mission in life. She had been an outstanding teacher for more than 30 years. Teaching was her life. She defined her worth as a person within the context of teaching. She felt God had called her to teach.

Karen's pastor helped her realize that she had defined her mission too narrowly. His questioning and thoughtful listening helped Karen redefine her mission more broadly, as giving love. One of the ways she did that as a teacher was by appreciating the value in each of her students and nurturing individuals by pointing out their values to them.

**Finding Options**: Her pastor suggested that until she could return to teaching she should find another way to fulfill her mission. Karen made a list of as many friends as she could think of. Then she wrote next to each name something she appreciated about that person.

**Taking Action**: She occupied her time each day by calling or writing friends to express this appreciation and love. In turn, she received calls and letters from them, expressing their appreciation for her friendship.

**Evaluating**: Her depression lifted, and she experienced the peace and contentment that comes when a person knows she is fulfilling her mission in life.

As problems become more complex, their resolution does also. Rather than follow a simple step-by-step problem-solving formula, complex problems weave back and forth from step 2 or 3 back to step 1. This reinforces the whole concept that life is a process, a journey that takes us in many directions. In Dan's case, he gained greater insight into his problem. He discovered more options as he moved forward in the process. He gained confidence about his ability to manage his life.

Bob became aware of his tendency to shift blame. In the process of solving his problems, he began to take responsibility for his problems.

Marie had had the opposite tendency from Bob, that is, taking on the entire burden of her problems and not seeking help. In discovering options that involved help from other people, her doctor, and physical therapist, she realized how alone she had felt. And she discovered how gratifying it is to feel supported.

Karen's problem solving led her on a spiritual journey of rediscovering the mission for her life.

In all cases, these people were able to make progress because they took action.

> To reach the port of heaven we must sail,
> sometimes with the wind and sometimes against it,
> but we must sail, not drift or lie at anchor.
>
> —Oliver Wendell Holmes

## Summary

- Knowing why a particular goal is important will reinforce your commitment to solving problems that get in your way.

- The person with a desire to find solutions will; the person without that desire will find excuses not to solve a problem.

- Determination is the strength and energy you put into finding solutions, trying them, and evaluating them.

- Perseverance is the duration of your effort, the ability to stick to it until the problem is solved.

- Start out by defining your problem, being accurate and specific. Avoid vagueness and generalities.

- List all the things you can do about your problem, brain-storming with a support group or your medical team.

- Take action on each of the solutions that seem appropriate. Give it an honest chance and then evaluate the situation to see if your problem is solved. If not, try another solution. Only action will move you ahead.

- When trying to solve a problem, deal first with any emotion it arouses until you can view the problem from a logical perspective.

## Reflection Questions

1. What is the major problem reducing your sense of well-being? State your problem accurately, specifically, and honestly, breaking it down if it is complex.


2. Describe why you want to solve your problem.


3. List all the ideas you can think of to solve your problem. (Make a long list, including even the "wild" ideas.)


4. Select the solutions that appeal most to you and list them.


5. Act on one of the options listed in #4.


Evaluate your action periodically. If the problem is solved, go on to another problem. If the problem is not solved, try another option from #4.

# Getting the Support You Need

One day I had lunch with a friend of mine who has arthritis. When her coffee was served to her she reached for a container of cream, set it in front of me, and asked simply: "Will you please open this for me?" The tone of her voice was matter-of-fact. With neither fanfare nor fuss, support was requested and given; a need was met.

Sometimes friends initiate the discussion about support, asking how they can give it. A blind friend of mine was delighted with the way one of her friends expressed this: "Don't let me do anything 'dorky.'" But other friends may not know whether you want help or how much to give; and they may feel awkward about asking. So you must be direct and explicit in explaining your needs to them.

Getting the support you need is a never-ending process, but once you understand and become good at techniques for helping others to help you, it becomes a natural and enriching part of a healthy life.

Support is as basic a need to human beings as is a strong foundation to a tall building. Knowing that your loved ones love you is part of that support. Feeling accepted by your friends and coworkers is supportive. Receiving help at a time of need is the kind of support that has woven the very fabric of humanity. It is support that gives people strength to cope with the many challenges of life.

The necessity of mutual support was well understood by the pioneers who settled North America. They got together frequently with neighbors to work, worship, and socialize. Each positive gathering affirmed their feeling of support and strengthened them individually and collectively.

Desperate, tragic challenges confronted them. Fire destroyed homes, barns, livestock, and crops. Weather and insects ruined crops some years. Disease hit and people died: old people, fathers, mothers, children. The long, harsh winters frustrated and isolated people. In fact, the sheer isolation drove some poor souls to madness. When the only teacher moved away, suddenly there was no one to teach school. The miracle is that people survived at all. Most important, and the message we can learn most from, is that they survived not only physically, but emotionally, psychologically, and spiritually as well. In fact, many became stronger, wiser, and more thankful than ever for all they had.

Like the pioneers, we also experience challenges, trials, and even tragedies. They survived and even thrived. So can we. Support helped them, and support can help us. In fact, the pioneers made use of all the life skills discussed in this book. They adapted, coped, solved problems, believed in a better tomorrow, used music and dancing to relieve stress, found motivation to get going, and nurtured the support they needed to keep going.

In working with people from rural areas, I have seen in them evidence of the pioneer spirit of our ancestors. I see two qualities that enhance their ability to survive—practicality and faith. They still face some of the challenges faced by the early pioneers: crop failure, loss of livestock due to disease, the windswept loneliness inherent to prairie life. But, like the pioneers of long ago, these are people who survive.

We can learn from these pioneers about support. Although challenges and circumstances change, the sources of support remain remarkably constant: family, friends, community, medical help (be that witchdoctor or MD), and a spiritual power.

This chapter will cover four of those basic sources of support: family, friends, community (this includes neighbors, coworkers, and members of groups to which you belong), and medical. Spiritual support is covered in the next chapter.

As these various sources of support are discussed, reflect upon the support you currently have. Identify areas of support you would like to strengthen. The chapter will also discuss specific techniques you can use to get that support.

**Medical support**

When you are diagnosed with a medical problem, your first supporters will be your medical team. The word "team" may not be familiar to you in describing your medical support. It describes all the people with whom you work to face your health challenge. Depending on your disease or disability, your team may include doctors, nurses, dietitians, counselors, secretaries, physical therapists, social workers, and anybody who works with you in some aspect of your well-being.

Chronic means "marked by long duration." People with chronic health problems face their challenges every day, for a long time. Since it is impractical to confer with one's doctor every day, the person with a health challenge must be knowledgeable enough to make many day-to-day decisions. That knowledge can come from your medical team as you participate with them in making decisions about your health. This means you are an important part of the team. Ultimately, *you* must take charge of the day-to-day decisions and maintenance of your health and well-being.

Now, let's examine the role of the medical team in promoting your well-being. As various aspects of medical support are described, identify the support you want but feel you are lacking.

The most obvious support from a medical team is the traditional role they play as medical experts. To receive the best advice, you need a physician who is knowledgeable in your specific health challenge. An endocrinologist is a specialist in diabetes, a cardiologist in heart disease, a rheumatologist in arthritis and lupus, an oncologist in cancer. Make certain that your team is led by a thoroughly knowledgeable specialist in your area. If you choose a generalist such as a family practitioner or an internist, find out how equipped that person is to manage your case. Some indicators of this might include: How many other patients with your disease this physician treats; with whom he or she affiliates; whether the person remains current by reading and attending medical seminars; whether he or she refers to specialists in your health challenge. From a knowledgeable medical team you can receive the support of excellent, up-to-date treatment.

The second form of support you can receive from your medical team is a comprehensive education in how to live well with your health challenge. Each member of the team has a unique and important message for you.

The medical team can also help you *problem solve.* That is, of course, help you to find your own solutions, not solve the problems for you. This works best for you if you inform the appropriate member of the team about a particular problem you may be having. That person and perhaps others on the team then brainstorm solutions with you, and then you choose the solution that appeals to you.

To the person with hypertension who says she's having trouble restricting salt, a dietitian might suggest specific low-sodium products, several cookbooks, and a low-salt cooking class.

To the cancer patient who feels his family is treating him as if cancer is contagious, a counselor might recommend some excellent books on cancer, a well-run local support group that offers both information and support for patients and families, or even an appointment with the family for them to express concerns directly to the doctor.

Here is an example of team problem solving I heard recently: A man with a heart problem told his dietitian that he felt genuinely depressed at the thought of having to restrict eating to accommodate a "heart healthy meal plan." The dietitian got details from him about the food he likes, the work day and weekend lifestyle patterns, and she even had him bring in menus from his favorite restaurants. Together they worked out a plan which contributed to the health of both his heart and his spirit. He found the energy and commitment to work on the physical issues when he became convinced that it was still possible to enjoy life.

The members of your medical team can also give support by being good role models. It is difficult to take advice to stop smoking from a physician who smokes. And it is inspiring and helpful when the physician who advises exercise is a regular exerciser. And the dietitian who eats the same way she tells me to eat truly convinces me that the diet recommended for people with diabetes is an excellent, healthy way for everyone to eat.

The communication of genuine caring is another way the medical team gives support. In the medical world they refer to the art versus the science of medicine. Knowledge and skill represent the science, while caring and person-to-person relating demonstrate the art. In all the years I have been a consumer of medical services, I have come to view caring as:

1. *Listening.* Real, honest-to-goodness attentiveness, eye-contact, facial response, question-asking, unfeigned interest, unhurried listening.

2. *Touching.* Genuine, laying-on-of-the-hands, I-care-about-you, you're-worthy-of-my-involvement touch.

3. *Responding.* Timely returned phone calls, complete answers to questions, a smile, a handshake or a hug, a caring one-human-being-to-another responsiveness.

The health care provider who communicates *positive expectations* supports hope in clients by giving the message, "I see positive energies in you. I know you can handle this." The German poet and philosopher Goethe expressed this when he said:

When we treat a man as he is, we make him worse than he is.
When we treat him as if he already were what he potentially could be, we make him what he should be.

Numerous studies have shown that people rise or fall to meet the expectations of the influential people in their lives. The health care provider who is upbeat and positive about your future promotes well-being in you rather than illness.

Blessed is the person whose medical team takes a wellness approach to the management of the health challenge. This is the best of three basic approaches: illness, prevention, and wellness.

These different approaches can be placed on a wellness continuum that goes from minus 100 to plus 100.


-100 . . . . . . . . . . . . . . . . . . . 0 . . . . . . . . . . . . . . . . . . . . . . +100
**Illness**                 **Prevention**               **Wellness**

The *illness* approach goes from -100 to 0 and is characterized by negative expressions like, "Since you have this disease you can expect the following deterioration of your health until you die." With this approach you wait until problems appear, then fix whatever can be fixed.

The *prevention* approach is right at 0 and encourages clients to have regular check-ups to catch problems as early as possible. Clients are taught what causes health problems and are encouraged to pursue behaviors designed to prevent them.

The *wellness* approach expands from 0 to +100 and encourages people to take care of themselves so they can continue to live a happy, fulfilling life. This approach is characterized by the positive expectation of an enriching future. This approach has been extremely important to me. The illness approach is out of the question for me, but I can't imagine taking the prevention approach either. I can't see myself getting out of bed in the morning, stretching, and saying, "Well, another day to prevent blindness and kidney failure!" As if that were a reason to live! It is the wellness approach to my diabetes that causes me to take insulin, test my blood sugar four times a day, exercise, and follow a prescribed meal plan so I feel well enough to enjoy my family, friends, and work.

My wonderful (carefully selected), wellness-oriented physician encourages my own wellness approach by asking questions about my life when we have appointments. She does not simply dwell on blood sugars and other physical aspects of my diabetes. This reinforces my own belief that I work hard to manage my diabetes so I can enjoy life, not simply prevent problems. This also reinforces my hope that I can prevent complications of the disease.

Your medical team members can help you learn helpful information, apply it to your health situation, and evaluate the results on your well-being. They should be viewed as an ongoing source of support.

## Encouraging medical support

Communication and cooperation are the basic ways in which we get the support we need from our medical team. The "Plan of Action" in the last chapter will serve as a good guide for your communication with your medical team.

Basically, discuss the goal(s) of your treatment plan with your medical team and reach agreement on how those goals will affect your well-being. Then, honestly and openly discuss the obstacles you will have to overcome to achieve those goals. That's where problem solving comes in. With your medical team's expertise and experience and your knowledge of your own capabilities, you can find ways to overcome your obstacles. Finally, let them know what you need for ongoing support (frequency of follow-up appointments, a phone call three days after beginning a new drug, etc.).

One of the best ways in which people can be cooperative members of their medical team is to become educated about their health challenge. We are all responsible for taking charge of our own well-being. We do that by seeking information, getting help understanding and applying the information to our own situation when necessary, and then making appropriate use of that information. To make the most of this process, you need to use assertiveness techniques to ask questions whenever you are unclear about something.

> Once when I had tendonitis, I went to an internist. He advised me to take cortisone. Fortunately, I had heard that cortisone can cause diabetes to be more difficult to manage. So I asked the internist, "What about my diabetes?" He looked startled and asked, "What diabetes?" Although my chart was right in front of him, he had not noticed that I have insulin-dependent diabetes. He then prescribed a different drug, but I would have had problems if I had not spoken up.

Another aspect of a cooperative attitude is to realize that anyone can make a mistake. I believe one of the reasons people are not more assertive with medical professionals is that they feel they are somehow superhuman. They aren't. They make mistakes just as you and I do. We must not view them as gods, nor should we view them as enemies. Take the attitude that we are all in it together.

We cannot expect our medical team to promote our health and well-being without our help. We must take responsibility as well by asking questions when we do not understand, or by asking the reason for something they have recommended. They certainly ought to be able to answer our questions in language we can understand and justify their recommendations in terms of our treatment goals. In order to nurture a relationship of mutual respect and trust, learn how to ask your questions in an assertive manner and not in an aggressive or passive manner. We will explore these three styles again later in the chapter, but here are some descriptions and examples of these varying communication styles in a medical context:

| | |
|---|---|
| Aggressive: | When I think only of myself. |
| Passive: | When I think only of the other person. |
| Assertive: | When I think of both of us. |

Let's apply each style to a specific situation:

Martha was in the hospital and at regular intervals she was given two pills. Her doctor had explained what the drugs were, how often they were to be taken, and what effect they might be expected to have. One evening the nurse brought her the pill cup and inside Martha saw the two familiar pills and a third pill she did not recognize.

The *aggressive* approach to this situation might be: "What's that third pill? What's wrong with this hospital anyhow? Are you trying to kill me?"

The *passive* approach would be to say nothing and simply take the pill, thinking, "I wonder what that third pill is? Oh well, they know best."

The *assertive* approach is simply to ask, "I recognize the iron pill and the benedryl, but what is the third pill?"

The most dramatic example of my needing to assert myself occurred shortly before I was to be married. My physician told me that he thought it was fine if I got married, "But don't have children," he said. "Don't spread your genes around." Instead of simply taking his advice, I chose to go with my husband to a genetic counselor. He gave us facts that were extremely encouraging. Then, based on real information, my husband and I made the choice to have a child. The supportive medical team I chose to see me through my pregnancy did not include the ill-informed and thoughtless physician who advised me not to have children.

Keep in mind that medical professionals are consultants. They can be hired and fired. This is not to suggest that we should not believe what medical professionals tell us. It does mean that we must filter all of what we are told and make our own educated, as well as intuitive, selection of what to believe.

## Family Support

Families are frequently a strong source of support. When one family member is in need, the whole family rallies to the aid of that person. The strongest demonstration of support usually occurs at the initial diagnosis of the disease. Family members are attentive, encouraging, helpful. Quite commonly, however, this support falls off with time. People once again become consumed by the challenges of their own lives and may withdraw from the active support they were giving to their family member in need.

By their very nature, chronic health challenges do not go away. What happens when the support is gone but the challenge stays? Naturally, different people have different experiences. Some report that their family support has never wavered; others feel a sense of loss of family support.

When we perceive a lack of support, we must look for ways to get support. But before you can ask for support, you must understand what you mean by support. For some it means a nonchalant attitude from family members; for others it means an intense involvement. For me it has been a combination of active support and simply ignoring my diabetes. I appreciate being treated like a "normal" person by my family, but I also appreciate their occasional recognition of my situation.

When we were children, my brother picked on me mercilessly, never treating me like anything but his "kid sister." Then, out of the blue, he would let me know he understood what I lived with.

When I was in ninth grade he was a senior in high school. One day he had to give a speech in English class on a subject of his choice. He chose to talk about diabetes. Like many ninth-graders, I was in awe of twelfth-graders. I was interested in what Pete would be telling his class about diabetes, because it seemed as though he would be saying it about me. I learned later that, among other things, Pete told the class "People with diabetes are actually better citizens because they have to be very well disciplined." Wow! My big brother said that about me! What tremendous support it was having that wonderful brother during those growing years.

My mother has certainly been the strongest, most consistent member in my support system. When I was first diagnosed, she made it seem that my diabetes was to be a blessing to our whole family. When I wanted to go to scout and church camps, Mother went along to work in the kitchen and pull weeds in the yard. She managed to achieve a perfect balance between providing me the support I needed without becoming overly protective and making me feel I'd never be able to make it without her. The only time I saw her was when I dashed over to her room to do my shot or when I passed through the cafeteria line and was "mysteriously" handed a plate with all the proper food exchanges. I knew someday I would be managing all that for myself, but I really appreciated her helping me with it then.

Mother's support took other forms once I left home. When I went away to college, she sent me the following poem:

> The rift in the chest of a mountain,
> The twist in the trunk of a tree,
> The water-cut cave in the hollow,
> The rough, rocky rim of the sea...
> Each one has a scar of distortion,
> Yet each has this sermon to sing,
> "The presence of what would deface me,
> Has made me a beautiful thing."

What loving, nurturing support from a mother to a daughter! Years later, it was to sustain me even more when my precious baby was injured and I helped him to accept his scars.

The support I receive from my husband and son is similar in that they are casual but concerned. We have worked out a system with which we are all comfortable. It works for all of us. When my blood sugar is low and my disposition suffers, my son has learned to leave me alone until my blood sugar becomes normal. And, when he has his moments of crankiness, I've learned to give him a bit of breathing room and time to get back into balance.

Reflect on the ways in which your family supports you. Think, too, of the ways in which you wish they were more supportive. For now, identify these two aspects of family support.

## Social support

Most of the people outside of our family come under the category of "social supports." They include neighbors, coworkers, fellow members of organizations, and, the most important of the social supports, friends.

When our son was six years old, he was faced with a major operation. The surgeon wanted to operate before John turned seven or eight. We sought advice from John's pediatrician on the timing of John's surgery with respect to his total well-being. We wanted to know not only when would be a good time in terms of physical considerations, but also in terms of John's psychological and emotional well-being. His response was, "Tell me about John's social supports. How does he feel about school? Does he have friends with whom he enjoys some good, imaginative play? Does he have good buddies? He'll be out of commission for awhile. Are his friends flakey, or are they the sort who will be there ready to play as soon as John's ready? My chief concern is social support."

The scientific community has studied the impact of social support and has reached the same conclusion our grandmothers did:

**Friends are an important part of a healthy, happy life.**

A friend told me this story about a little boy who came home later than expected one day. His mother asked him where he'd been. He said, "Well, Billy's bike broke down, so I had to help him."

His surprised mother said, "I didn't know you knew how to fix bikes."

"I don't," he said, "but I could help him cry."

Not only do people enjoy friendships on a daily basis, they also derive great support from knowing they have the kind of friends who will *be there* if needed.

Besides the specific support your friends can offer you, how would you characterize your social support needs? It is important that you define those needs so that you can start working to fill them. Here is how people I have met have described the support they want from friends. *Explore* their descriptions. *Reflect* on the kind of support you want.

**Listening:** I always feel "listened to" when I'm with my friends. That makes me feel better.

**Patience:** They know my limitations and my needs. They never make me feel like a burden but help me fill my needs matter-of-factly.

**Respect:** They are ready to give physical assistance only when I ask for it.

**Inspiration**: They've made it successfully through either the same challenge or one similar in magnitude.

**Distraction**: They're always ready for fun and laughter. I can count on these friends to help me get my mind off my troubles.

**Acceptance**: They don't judge me; they make me feel loved and cared about "no matter what."

**Cheerfulness:**They're generally upbeat.They're optimistic people, and just being with them or talking with them on the phone gives me a boost.

**Guidance:** They love me enough to speak to me honestly. They don't let me get away with feeling sorry for myself and getting stuck in self-pity. They help point me in a positive direction.

Now, *evaluate.* Of these descriptions, are there some that tell you how you'd like to get support from friends? Use them as a means to identify what you are looking for from each of your friends. It is perhaps a more serious friend who will prove to be an excellent listener. Your cheerful, upbeat friend may not be as good a listener, but you value him or her for lifting your spirits.

Also evaluate the way in which you ask for support. Would you want to support someone who asks the way you do? A sure way to turn off your supporters is to be whiney, demanding, or constantly negative. People have a tendency to finally stop asking, "How are you?" when the only response they ever get is negative. Listen to and observe yourself. Do you expect friends and family to read your mind? They can't. Communicate your needs.

If you feel that the friends you now have cannot meet all your social support needs, you may want to get involved in clubs or organizations in which you can meet new friends. Remember that social support is a two-way street, and that to get the depth of support you need, you must be able to give support. For example, if you are a good listener, try asking a new friend to tell you about his or her life; it could be the start of a deep, trusting friendship.

Be open to receiving support from people you have not yet met. I received tremendous support from just such a friend.

A woman I knew died suddenly after what seemed to be a victorious recovery from a kidney transplant. Stephanie was in her twenties. Those of us who had been through even a part of her struggle were stunned by her death. We thought that after all the trial and difficulty she had finally made it. Her funeral was particularly sad and I wept throughout it. I reflected upon what seemed an intolerable injustice. Stephanie had suffered terribly before and throughout her transplant. She wanted so desperately to live. She had made it through the transplant and was recovering beautifully. Then, suddenly, she was gone.

I felt numb as I left the church following the funeral. As I walked down the street to my car, I was greeted by a friend. I turned and saw that she was with a Laotian woman whom our church sponsors. The Laotian woman was very new to our country and spoke no English. I felt a bit awkward because of my tears. I explained to my friend that I had been to a funeral. Then, I looked at the other woman. I gestured toward the church, then helplessly looked back at her, trying to explain. As I looked into her face, I saw my anguish mirrored in her eyes. She knew. Not only did she know that I was grieving for a friend, but she herself *knew* the same anguish. She had lost young friends in Laos. She had, in fact, left her mother and eldest son in Laos. She knew sadness, injustice, and she also knew peace.

That brief, wordless encounter began my healing. Although Stephanie's death still seems an injustice, I derived a small bit of peace when I realized that people do survive injustice. I felt connected with another human being who understood my pain, because she had also struggled with pain and had come to her own peace.

Identify *who* your social supports are and *how* they fill your support needs.

## Encouraging family and social support

In order to receive support, you usually need to ask for it. You have defined the support you need or want, and now the next step is to actively seek it. Sometimes it is difficult to ask for support. Our culture encourages self-reliance and independence. People must work at being "interdependent." A healthy life is a balance of independence and dependence; sometimes I need you and sometimes you need me. That's interdependence and that's healthy.

**Mutual respect** is the foundation from which family and social support arise. Interdependence comes out of mutual respect. It is an even larger issue of basic respect for life. It is an expression of the shared value of a fulfilling life, a recognition that a problem has placed that value in jeopardy, and a request for help from one human being to another.

**Giving support** naturally follows mutual respect. Look for opportunities to give support to the people from whom you would like to receive it. You can set the "tone" of a relationship through your spirit and acts of giving. Sending a pot of soup to a neighbor who has a house full of out-of-town guests is the sort of act that encourages a phone call or visit when you need it.

**Gratitude,** expressed in a simple, sincere "Thank you!" is the cement that binds relationships. This positive reinforcement of positive behavior makes it more likely that the person will offer it again. Buy a stack of thank you post cards and postage stamps so you're always ready. Reinforce every kindness with a thank you. Remember to express gratitude to your family, for they are most often neglected or taken for granted. Some people report that one of the positive aspects of their disease is the appreciation and expressions of love and gratitude it fostered among family members.

**Communication** is vital to the development of supportive relationships. We will examine three areas in communication: education, assertiveness, and listening.

Education of family members encourages cooperation (eating meals on time), alleviates or removes fear ("Nothing in life is to be feared. It is only to be understood." [Marie Curie]), and promotes understanding. ("So that's why you feel like that after chemotherapy!") Friends whom you've educated can give you the sort of support that removes obstacles. When our friends invite us to dinner they let me know what they'll be serving and what time it will be served. They understand I need information to plan for my insulin needs. How supportive that is!

Assertiveness is defined in *Your Perfect Right* by Robert Alberti and Michael E. Emmons as:

> Behavior which enables a person to act in his/her own best interests, to stand up for him/herself without undue anxiety, to express his/her honest feelings comfortably or to exercise his/her rights without denying the rights of others.

Unassertiveness creates unnecessary pain, and problems. For example, when a person with poor mobility neglects to tell friends, she may be forced to climb many stairs rather than be a burden. When a person with digestive problems eats whatever is served for fear of being impolite, he may become ill later. Let your friends know what you need and why you need it. Keep interdependence in mind.

If you find yourself feeling uncomfortable about asking for what you need, imagine that the situation is reversed. Imagine your best friend has the disease or special requirement. Wouldn't you, as a friend, want to do everything you could to be supportive? Wouldn't you feel hurt if you found out your friend had a special dietary need and had not told you when he or she ate at your home?

Whole books have been written on assertiveness. If you feel a special need to get help in this area, seek books and classes that teach assertiveness. Here are the basic guidelines to keep in mind.

1. Enter into assertive behavior only after giving yourself positive messages so that your attitude is positive. One such message is the definition by Alberti and Emmons. Review it before expressing yourself.

2. Practice being assertive. Like any skill, it won't come overnight. Practice in nonthreatening situations with people you feel comfortable with. For example, a woman with diabetes disliked the way her mother-in-law ceremoniously served her sugar-free gelatin. Practicing with her husband, she came up with this message: "Joan, it was very thoughtful of you to make me sugar-free gelatin. Thank you. But I feel embarrassed when you announce it at the table. Could we please just be casual about it?"

3. Be factual instead of emotional. You can talk about your feelings in a factual manner. Tone of voice (calm rather than whiney) helps you to keep the discussion factual. "I feel lonely when you never ask me how I'm getting along. When you know that I've been to the doctor, I would feel so supported if you remembered that and inquired about it."

4. Rehearse it. Visualize yourself looking calm and in charge, then plan what you want to say. Find a quiet spot somewhere, where you can actually rehearse it.

Listening is the other half of communication. What are your family's and friends' needs? Are they frightened by your disease or disability? Deal with that through education, taking them with you to one of your doctor visits or to a counseling session. Listen to their general needs. Surely the disease or disability has become a part of both your family and social life, and as such, it must be dealt with. But your family and friends still have their own needs that have nothing to do with your challenge.

It may be difficult to seriously consider your daughter's acne or a friend's broken car when you feel that your challenge is so much greater. Try to see their problems for what they are: problems in need of solutions. Explain to them the steps in the solution-finding chapter. In doing that you will have participated in mutual support. You will have risen above your illness to deal with the needs of another person, which can help you to experience a feeling of emotional well-being.

Some friends will be more supportive than others. You can choose to gravitate toward those who support you. But because you live with family members day in and day out, it is crucial to have their support. If you find that you and your family are simply unable to follow these guidelines to establish a healthy system of communication, then do seek help. Family counseling is a wise step in a very healthy direction.

It will take time for family counseling to help. I once heard someone say, "Oh, it isn't worth it. It'll probably take a year for us to iron out all our problems!" Ask yourself this: In one year would you prefer to have a healed and healthy family because you spent that year in counseling, or would you prefer to still be in a broken or unhealthy family? Support comes in many forms, and counseling is one. Healthy people get the support they need.

## Support groups

A support group is people who face a similar problem and are willing to share their successes and failures in dealing with it. These are people whom you do not have to educate or encourage to support you, for they are organized to provide social support and problem-solving discussions. Support groups are usually led by a counselor or other medical professional, or they may be led by clergy or a layperson who has been trained to lead a support group. If a group is made up of people who are living well with their challenge, it can provide the additional support of inspiration. But if you find you've joined a group made up of poor copers who enjoy complaining, it can reinforce your problems instead of solving them. If you decide to join a support group, ask your medical team to recommend one that is reputable and well-run.

There are options for the format of support groups. Some groups prefer to be purely supportive in the sense of providing a forum where people can come and express themselves. At each meeting people share what has happened in their life since the last time the group met. People with urgent needs can request a first "hearing."

Another format is similar to the problem-solving approach: identify the problem, list your options, choose an option, and act. Some people prefer this format because they get suggestions from the others on solutions. The third format includes a speaker; this, then, combines education and support. The philosophy for a group can be expressed in a simple creed: "We will accept one another, listen to one another, and care about one another. We will grow." Groups can be kept "on track" by reviewing the format and philosophy at the beginning of each meeting.

Here is a practical suggestion for assessing your support. Draw a circle and write your name in it. Then draw lines radiating out from the circle forming "spokes." At the end of each line write the name of a person, an organization, or elements of your life that support you. Next to the names of your supporters, describe how they support you. Once you have identified supporters and the type of support they give you, then you are in a good position to ask for the additional support you want.

Here is an example of my wheel of support for my diabetes.

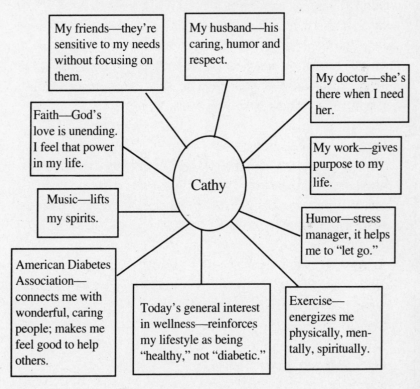

Do your wheel and refer back to it from time to time, especially when you are feeling in need of more support. Are there new supporters? Has some of the support you want diminished or stopped? How can you get it again?

Since your disease is only part of your life, consider the support you need for all the other areas. Think of your life as composed of a series of roles. Each of us plays a variety of roles in a lifetime: employee, spouse, parent, child, sibling, and such wonderfully diverse roles as artist, volunteer, gourmet cook, athlete, and musician.

Do a wheel of support for each of your roles. A satisfying life requires that the roles we value are fulfilled to the best of our ability. Our various roles weave together to make the colorful fabric we call our life.

Ultimately, the support you need goes beyond the physical and the psychological to the spiritual. The next chapter turns to the spiritual force in your life, your Physician Within. We will look at nourishing that force.

> If I had but three loaves of bread,
> I would sell one and buy hyacinths,
> For they would feed my soul.
> —The Koran

Before we can nourish that force, we must discover it.

## Summary

Support from others is as basic a need to human beings as a strong foundation is to a tall building.

- Your basic sources of support are family, friends and other social acquaintances, and the members of your medical team.

- Successful management of most chronic health challenges requires a knowledgeable and coordinated medical team, each of whom can teach you about a specific part of your health needs and help you solve problems related to those needs. Your team supports you, further, by being good role models and by communicating genuine caring.

- Management of a health challenge can be characterized by one of three basic approaches: Illness, in which you wait for problems to appear and try to fix what can be fixed; prevention, in which you have check-ups to try to catch things as early as possible and in which you follow specific behaviors because they may prevent problems; and wellness, in which you take care of yourself so you can live a happy, fulfilling life.

- To encourage your medical team to support you, nurture a sense of mutual respect, give support to others, discuss with them your treatment goals, any obstacles you'll need to overcome; then let them know what you need for ongoing support.

- Communicate your needs using an assertive manner.

Assertiveness is thinking of yourself and the person with whom you are communicating; it is telling someone what you need and why; it is asking questions or requesting an explanation, realizing that anyone can make a mistake.

- Before you can ask for support from your family you must decide how you would like to be supported, whether casually or intensely, or somewhere in between.

- Friends can provide different types of support, depending on whether each is a good listener, an inspiring example, or a cheerful spirit-lifter. Likewise, you can provide support through your personality strengths. By giving support, you will be more likely to get support from friends.

- Seek out a professional counselor or a support group to amplify the support you get from your family and friends.

## Reflection Questions

1. Describe how you want to be supported by your

   Medical team

   Friends

   Family

   Others

2. Write out specific actions you will take to encourage more support in your life.

3. List ways you will give support to those sources of support.

4. Draw a wheel of support—a circle with your name in it and lines radiating out from the circle to a name, organization, or element in your life that supports you.

# Discover Your Physician Within

A challenge to one's well-being may bring greater rewards than wealth, possessions, and power. Pain and disease can actually teach self-discovery and can result in growth. People have reported feeling grateful for suffering, for example, because through it they gained self-esteem, insight, and integrity. Facing serious illness or death, many learn to identify and concentrate on the things that matter most to them. As these persons draw on the gifts of the spirit, they find that the material world gives way to the spiritual, and they experience love, peace, joy, and hope.

Unlike those with a rich spiritual life, who readily integrate their spirit into every experience, those without one may ask life's most profound questions only when faced with a great health challenge. And these kinds of questions will naturally lead to the spiritual domain. This kind of soul searching reminds us that we will not live forever—a fact we've always known intellectually. But when we learn it with our heart, it can be distressing. To live comfortably with the fact of our mortality, we turn to the spiritual.

In this chapter, you will be encouraged to examine the spiritual component of your life. How do you describe it? How does it support you? How do you nourish it? How do you connect with it? When you know the answers to these questions, you will have discovered your Physician Within.

Your Physician Within is that force which you recognize as being greater than you are. No one can define it for you or describe what it will mean in your life. In this chapter, I will share with you some of the discoveries others have made, as well as my personal understanding of my Physician Within. But you must look into your own soul and discover that powerful, essential force that lies within *you*.

Once you identify this force you need to figure out how to *activate* and *nourish* it. Although this power source can be a person's most important support, many individuals ignore it and don't completely understand it. It is fairly easy for us to identify our external sources of support: family, spouse, friends, doctor, pastor, counselor, etc. But our internal source of support is not visible. You can feel its strength and support but you cannot see it. It is difficult for us to believe in something we cannot see. That is your greatest challenge, because it is *faith* that activates your Physician Within.

We know that there is more to human beings than body and mind. There is also spirit. The more organized and concrete resources for studying the spirit include philosophy, literature, and religion. The most convincing resource, however, is experience. Sometimes we experience spirituality by observing others, and this can be convincing and helpful. But your own direct, personal experience will be the most persuasive and valuable means of discovering your Physician Within.

Many experiences can contribute to your belief in this force, but often life's darkest, most difficult moments help us to discover and fully appreciate this wonderful, sustaining, never-ending source of strength and comfort.

When our precious son was born, I had had diabetes for 19 years. It was still the "Dark Ages" of diabetes management, in that blood glucose monitoring was not yet available to allow close control of blood glucose on a daily basis. So my diabetes was not easily managed, and the pregnancy was in the high-risk category, unlike today.

Thankfully, our son was born triumphantly healthy. However, he became the victim of a hospital mistake. He was slightly low in calcium at birth, and an IV solution of calcium was delivered at ten times the prescribed concentration. Our newborn was seriously burned. He lost all the skin, fatty tissue, veins, and some of the nerves from his knee to his toes on one leg. A plastic surgeon performed split-thickness skin grafting, and John finally came home at age four weeks.

For several months our life centered around our precious baby and the ongoing challenge of his injury. Although the skin graft was successful, it was contracting as it healed. His foot was being pulled up. We took him to an orthopedic surgeon, who applied a new plaster cast to his leg each week. As the plaster dried, the surgeon applied great pressure downward so that the hardened cast would hold John's foot down. As one of the first casts was removed, we discovered that John's leg was swollen with a terrible infection. The graft had not healed enough to be covered with a plaster cast. The pediatrician ordered X-rays, and we waited in anguish to learn whether the infection had invaded the bone. Thankfully, it hadn't.

It was a difficult time for us, waiting for this nightmare to end. One problem after another surfaced. And although our attention was focused on John, other concerns arose. My husband Dale, a teacher, was aware that his school was facing severe budget cuts; there was talk of layoffs. We didn't worry about these "might be's." We had enough real problems demanding our attention.

During times of difficulty we find comfort in being able to talk with people in our support system. But for the first time in my life, I felt I couldn't go to my friends and family. Although they loved and supported us in general, they could not support our decision not to sue the hospital. One acquaintance even told me that I was a bad mother for not suing. She thought I ought to be concerned about providing for John's future through a cash settlement. We were concerned about John's future, but we would provide for his needs on our own.

Finally, we retreated from our support network and drew in toward our little family of three. We concentrated on doing what we had to do for John. The next decision was to put a fiberglass cast on his leg and leave a window over the graft area so that we could dress it and air could get to it. It was heavy and cumbersome. John couldn't lie down to sleep, so we placed him in his infant seat in his crib. He cried endlessly. I kept telling myself that he wasn't in pain, that he was just crying because of the awkwardness and the frustration of not being able to really stretch out.

After two weeks, this cast was removed. When it was cut off, I was horrified to discover a sadly misshapen little foot. The window cut-out had caused uneven pressure on John's foot and bent it grossly out of shape. My first thought was, "All that crying *was* from pain. My baby has suffered so much!" It was the lowest moment of my life; my heart broke. The surgeon shook his head and said, "We'll just leave casts off for a while now." I took John home.

When Dale got home that night I couldn't wait to unburden myself. The minute he walked through the door I began to tell of our dreadful experience and John's poor little foot. When I finally finished, I realized that my husband looked dazed. His first words were, "I lost my job today."

At that very instant, I knew we were going to be fine. I felt a strange peace settle over me, which in light of the circumstances surely transcended normal understanding. More important, I knew that a power greater than Dale and I was in control and would take care of us and our son.

My Physician Within is God. God is within me at all times, but for me to derive strength and help, I must first yield control of the situation to God.

That is not an easy thing to do normally. We each have our own comfort level with control, and I am most comfortable when I feel that *I* am in control. But, there are times when we have to let go because we are clearly not able to control what is happening. My husband was the youngest teacher in his department. That had been the single criterion for deciding which teacher to cut. We could not control that. Our baby had been the innocent victim of one of those classic, tragic mistakes—also totally beyond our control.

It is now 18 years since our baby was born. One of the insights I gained from that experience is a spiritual gift that guides me today. After turning control over to God, I felt the lifting of an enormous burden. And, along with the lifting of that burden, I experienced a continuation of peace and a strengthened faith.

Perhaps because of the long duration of John's therapies and treatments, I stayed in close touch with God through prayer and Bible reading and the blessing of friends who prayed for us. I got into the spiritual habit of daily and many times a day connecting with God. The surprising discovery was that God was there to help me with my daily life, no matter how mundane or trivial my concerns were. For me, the spiritual gift was the insight that I can place all my concerns in God's hands and receive direction for my life.

Because I'm human, I still snatch control back from time to time. But, because I still read the Bible and pray daily, I keep turning it back over to God. Realizing my human limitations and weaknesses has allowed me to understand what the Apostle Paul meant when he told the story of having a thorn in his side. He asked God three times to remove the thorn, but three times God refused to do so. God's response was, "My grace is sufficient for you. My power is made perfect in your weakness."

Look back on your life. Have you experienced that sort of inner peace and strength? Perhaps you have already defined your Physician Within. Once you have truly experienced the power of your internal support, you will be able to specifically define it and believe in it. Defining what you believe that spiritual force to be and what it means in your life is a necessary step toward gaining the most support in times of greatest need. Sharing that feeling and observing other's experiences with their spirituality will help you to further explore this beautiful and mysterious part of life.

History books and newspapers are filled with accounts of people who have survived horrible challenges to the body, mind, and spirit. Driven by a strong spiritual component, they picked themselves up and kept going. Even more inspiring than the experiences themselves is the realization that, despite great difficulty, these persons continue to survive and celebrate life.

**Who are your heroes?**

I have derived enormous strength and inspiration from my mother. When my baby was injured, I was able to give him the same strength and inspiration Mother so beautifully gave me when I was diagnosed with diabetes. Prior to John's second surgery, I clung to the memories of Mother's cheerfulness and positive conviction that everything would be fine. So with John I was full of laughter and play. We celebrated life. With family, friends, and pastor, however, I contemplated the precariousness of life. My questions brought tears instead of answers. I was afraid that perhaps I was too weak to be able to inspire my child the way Mother had inspired me.

It helped when I gained further insight into what Mother had faced and how she actually felt at that time. She always had seemed so upbeat, but she told me years later that when she practiced giving injections to an orange, tears streamed down her face as she imagined having to inject her little girl. That revelation amazed me because it was always a smiling and positive "sergeant of arms" (and legs and buttocks) who marched into my bedroom to give me my shot and start me on my healthy way each day. I thought it had been easy for Mother to be cheerful. I found it even more inspiring to learn that it was not easy at all, but she had done it.

Perhaps because of the environment in which he grew or perhaps on his own, John, with proverbial "childlike faith," discovered his Physician Within.

When John was three years old, the surgeon told us that he would need more surgery. The graft had contracted and pulled his foot up into a 90 degree angle. The surgeon solemnly told me that although he could graft enough skin to allow John to walk and run, John would never be able to completely flex his toes. "He'll never point his toes; there simply isn't enough skin," he told me.

This time the surgeon took a full thickness of skin from John's abdomen. When the stitches were removed, John's foot was in the exact position the surgeon had told us it would be. He reminded me, "Now, remember, that foot is not going to come down any farther. Creams won't help. Exercise won't help. He simply doesn't have enough skin."

We went home and got on with our lives. One day as John was riding his trike up a particularly steep hill, I pushed on his back to help him make it up. He looked at me and insisted, "Mom, I can do it myself." So I let go and followed alongside him. As he worked to get up the hill, he hoarsely whispered the words, "I think I can. I think I can. . ."

Several months later, we returned to the plastic surgeon for a check-up. He confirmed what we had already observed: John was able to point both toes perfectly. The surgeon's face registered real shock as he said, "There's no explanation for that!"

Ten days later, as John was getting out of the bathtub, I pointed to the graft donor site on his abdomen and said, "Isn't that super, John? Your scar is fading so that you can hardly see it." He looked me straight in the eyes and said, "Mom, my body's got lots of skin, and I'm healthy!" I told that story to a group once, and there happened to be a pediatric plastic surgeon in the audience. He approached me afterwards and told me he wasn't at all surprised at John's healing. He said children do not understand "never." They expect to get well. And they frequently do, in spite of all our doubts and learned realism.

There is something quite wonderful about childlike faith. Children's limited exposure to the world has not taught them hopelessness. They live in a magical world where anything is possible.

John taught me yet another lesson about faith when he was six years old. It was a warm spring day, and John came running to the front door to tell me that a baby robin had fallen from its nest. I responded by getting a cardboard box and filling it with leaves and grass. Then I got a medicine dropper and made a thin preparation of oatmeal (that's how we nurture baby birds back to health in Minnesota!) When John showed me the baby robin, I was horrified. It was far too premature to survive. At this point, John was jumping up and down, enthusiastically telling me that he had named the robin "Oscar." I felt miserable because I knew that the little robin couldn't possibly make it. I told John that we'd do the best we could for Oscar.

That night as John was preparing for bed, he told me he wanted to include Oscar in his prayers. I didn't know whether I should get into a discussion of how God always answers our prayers but not always the way we want them answered. But I decided not to discuss theology. We prayed. And Oscar made it. He grew to be a strong, healthy bird. And just before he flew away, he perched in the tree next to our garage where we got a photograph of him. That photograph is still on our refrigerator. We've replaced our refrigerator over the years, but that photo goes right back. I need it as a reminder to have faith. I need to remind myself that I don't know everything and that knowledge itself is limited.

Recall the stories in your life that have inspired you. Compare the experiences of others with your own, and enrich your appreciation of the power within each of us. Again, the most helpful resources for your discovery of your Physician Within will be your own intimate experience with difficulty, emotional pain, and all of life's challenges and seeming "unfairness," all of which, when overcome, add so much to the imperfect but beautiful reality of life.

The Physician Within can be God, a deeply held Conviction, Faith, Hope, Trust, Peace. Each of us uses a term that best describes the spirit that guides us. Philosophy, poetry, and religion are simply attempts to put all that into words. Inasmuch as these expressions of others' beliefs succeed in describing your beliefs, they reinforce and nourish your Physician Within. Let's explore ways of nourishing, reinforcing, and sustaining the Physician Within.

## Philosophy

To live comfortably with the fact of our mortality each of us becomes a philosopher. We choose a philosophy of life that gives us strength to live with the unwelcome knowledge that we are mortal.

Our philosophies frequently are expressed through favorite quotations that make tangible the intangible.

> To teach men how to live without certainty,
> and yet without being paralyzed by hesitation,
> is perhaps the chief thing philosophy can still do.
> —Bertrand Russell

The French philosopher Albert Camus made the following observation:

> In the depth of winter I finally learned that
> within me there lay an invincible summer.

I love that philosophical description of the Physician Within as "an invincible summer," especially in facing the "depth of winter." Life brings us many winters. A friend of mine lost her teenaged daughter in a car accident. She found strength from Camus' words because she could believe that her daughter, for all eternity, would remain in the spring of her life. A disease is one of life's winters. The force that keeps you going through the darkest hours of the harshest winter is your Physician Within.

## Literature

Hope is the thing with feathers that perches in the soul
And sings the tune without the words
And never stops at all.

—Emily Dickinson

One of my mentors reminded me that not *all* philosophy and literature is inspiring. Some of it is dark and disturbing. Here is where your responsibility comes in. Choose a nourishing food for your mind and soul just as you carefully select nourishing food for your body. As the German poet Goethe so beautifully put it:

One ought, every day at least, to hear a little song, read a good poem, see a fine picture, and, if it were possible, to speak a few reasonable words.

Here are two examples of simple, perhaps surprising thoughts from literature. The first is Willa Cather's.

Where there is great love, there are always miracles. Miracles rest not so much upon faces or voices or healing power coming to us from afar off, but on our perceptions being made finer, so that for a moment our eyes can see and our ears can hear what is there about us always.

—Willa Cather

The best things are nearest. Breath in your nostrils, Light in your eyes, Flowers at your feet, Duties at your hand, the Path of Right just before you. Then do not grasp at the stars, but do Life's plain, common work as it comes, certain that daily duties and daily bread are the sweetest things in life.

—Robert Louis Stevenson

Newspapers are not always full of the world's problems. The Wall Street Journal periodically has a full page sponsored by United Technologies Corporation, and rather than an advertisement, each page shares a stimulating thought. I saved the following one because it fired my spirit.

## Brighten Your Corner

Have you
noticed the
great difference
between the
people you meet?
Some are as
sunshiny as
a handful of
forget-me-knots.
Others come on
like frozen mackerel.
A cheery, comforting
nurse can

help make a
hospital stay
bearable.
An upbeat secretary
makes visitors
glad they came
to see you.
Every corner of the
world has its clouds,
gripes, complainers,
and pains in the
neck—because many
people have
yet to
learn that
honey works better
than vinegar.
You're in control
of your small
corner of the
world.
Brighten it. . .
You can.

## Religion

Millions of people find their greatest source of strength, power, and hope in their religious faith. Prayer, meditation, and worship nourish the spirit. Jewish and Christian traditions both encourage worship within their families of faith with prayers offered for those in need of healing. It is customary in the Jewish tradition to recite a Mi-She-Barakh in the synagogue. It is a prayer offered for those who are ill.

Similar counsel is found in the New Testament: "Is there any sick among you? Let him call the elders of the church and let them pray over him, anointing him with oil in the name of the Lord. And the prayer of faith shall save the sick. . ." (James 5:14). The following are prayers from the Christian and Jewish traditions.

> O Lord, may we have thy mind and thy spirit;
> make us instruments of thy peace;
> where there is hatred, let us sow love;
> where there is injury, pardon;
> where there is discord, union;
> where there is doubt, faith;
> where there is despair, hope;
> where there is darkness, light;
> and where there is sadness, joy.

O Divine Master, grant that we may not so much seek to be consoled as to console; to be understood, as to understand; to be loved, as to love; for it is in giving that we receive; it is in pardoning that we are pardoned; and it is in dying that we are born to eternal life.

—Saint Francis of Assissi

> God, hear all our prayers; the words and thoughts
> that pour forth, as well as "our sighs too deep for
> words." When we are alone it is easy to be afraid;
> be with us in our fears. May your promise, "Lo, I
> am with you always," fill our need to be close to you.
> We pray that your presence may be a blessing of
> peace and hope for the hours to come. God, hear
> all our prayers.

Unto Thee, O Lord do I call.
And unto Thee do I make supplication.
Hear O Lord and be gracious unto me;
O Lord, be Thou my Helper.
Thou healest the broken-hearted,
And bindest up their wounds.
Thou who has done great things,
O God, who is like Thee?
Hide not from me in the day of my distress:
Turn unto me and speedily answer my prayer.
Heal me, O Lord, and I shall be healed.
Save me and I shall be saved; for Thou art my
praise.

      (Psalm 30:10; 147:3; 71:19; 102:2,3; Jeremiah 17:14)

And the following meditation reflects yet another tradition—
Native American:

*An Indian Version of the Twenty-Third Psalm*

Father, guardian of earth and the heavens
Along with all things, I am your creation.
You are the tree of life; I am the branch.
Flowering, thankful, and contented.

The marvels, the natural elements you have made
I am in reverence and wonder about them.
Through your love and guidance, you give me
A precious vine to hold onto.
It is the thread of life to follow.
It leads me satisfied among the
Fragrant meadows and waters.

It is you who has provided
The fruits of life and I am happy.

You provide my sustenance, nourishment
From the land, the waters, and the air.
I am blessed. I give thanks for all.
I am satisfied. My bowl is plenty.

You are the Spirit at our center.
With you I am strong, my heart good.
Sometimes it is not easy, this life's road.
Sometimes I fall, tested. You give me
Strength and direction to carry on,
To pursue a path of goodness
and to care for others.

Life is but a part of the cycle
A beginning. As with all things in time
I know I must leave behind this
Earthly life entering another journey
That I shall travel with no fear—for
You are with me now, then, and forever.

Bad times come with the good, but good will prevail.
I speak from the heart. I have done my best
To follow the good path, ready for the next journey.
I am prepared. It is then, in the great heavenly lodge
Rejoining my relatives, with pride in a life liven,
That I will humbly present myself, Spirit Father,
     In heaven, as on earth forever.

                            —Nakoma

*For information on the beautiful nature and Native American art by Nakoma, write Nakoma, P.O. Box 1421, Rochester, MN 55903.*

How do you define and describe your Physician Within? If your discovery is still incomplete, then keep searching. Philosophy, literature, and religion can not only nourish and reinforce your spirit, they can also help you to discover it. Besides these resources, talk with advisors whom you respect: health professionals, clergy, educators, friends you admire, and any people you know who are "survivors" in the best sense of the word. They have made the best of what they've been given in life, be it poverty, injury, loss, or chronic disease. If you seek your spirit with the belief that you will find it—you will! Once you discover your Physician Within, you will realize that the power has been within you all along.

Remember, the only way in which we can activate the Physician Within is through faith...belief. It is so easy not to believe. Belief can be so fragile, while reality is often so bold and large and strong. A friend of mine was a guest in our home shortly before she died. When she was last in our home, she was a blind, kidney-transplanted, amputeed young woman. I helped her to prepare for her bath. As I lowered her frail little body into the bathtub, I grieved for her, but I also grieved for myself. Diabetes had caused all that devastation to her body. I have the same disease. Belief in health is difficult when the reality of disease is so strong. I remember quite vividly what it felt like to rub cream on the stump of her leg.

Reality's shrill voice can pierce to the core of our being. The Physician Within must be a powerful force in order to absorb that piercing cry and answer back with calm, sure, strength: "Yes, but I am in control. Trust. Believe."

I am convinced that disease and pain and difficulty can be blessings because of the spiritual growth they can bring. Without struggle, we remain weak. A perfect illustration of this comes from the story of a man who raised butterflies as a hobby. He was so touched by the difficulties they had in emerging from the cocoon, that once, out of mistaken kindness, he split a cocoon with his thumbnail so that the tiny inmate could escape without a struggle. That butterfly was never able to use its wings.

To find the strength to carry on with whatever struggle life brings, we need an unending source of inner power—our Physician Within. When we are unaware of that power, we are ignoring it. If suffering causes us to seek that force, then suffering is valuable. It is your responsibility to connect with your Physician Within. View it as a huge generating plant into which you must be "plugged" in order to make use of its energy and power. Use it or not; it is *your* choice. If you choose to connect with this power source, look for all the "sockets" you can plug yourself into. Receive all the spark it has to ignite your spirit.

## Sparks to ignite your spirit

Even with an active internal power, we are not towers of strength, acceptance, and peace all the time. There are times of honest questioning, times of vulnerability, momentary returns of anger and sadness over disease and disability. And there are simply days when we're "down." These are the times to turn—with the help of our Physician Within—to our external power sources and receive their spark.

## People

People can be wonderful sparks. This book is "peopled" by the brave men and women from my world as I have observed them and been inspired by them. Look for the inspiring people in your life. They're there.

One of my dearest friends has been an inspiring model to me all my life. Norma is 97 years old as this book is being written. During the Depression, Norma and her husband owned and managed a hotel. Harry became ill and required round-the-clock nursing care. Norma struggled to run the hotel by herself.

One day I asked Norma, "How did you make it?" She responded with the spirit of practicality and faith that I have admired in so many people. "Well, on days when I was feeling down, I'd think about someone worse off than I. Then, I'd go visit them. On days when I was really down, I'd go to a movie where I could escape for a couple of hours. Feeling refreshed, I would then visit someone in a nursing home or hospital. Then, I'd get on with my life."

## Nature

Nature is a magnificent spark! Have you ever looked so closely at a Norway pine tree that it stirred a feeling of inspiration in you? The Norway pine is tall, straight, strong, resolute, yet able to bend and sway with the wind. What a lesson can be learned from this beautiful, resilient tree!

Birds inspire me. One April we had a blizzard in Minnesota. The robins in our neighborhood had already arrived and built their nests, but the blizzard destroyed them. I saw that the robins didn't give up. They rebuilt their nests with resilience and determination!

The physical environment surrounding us can have a dramatic effect on how we feel and view our life situation. Researchers have focused extensively on the sunlight's effect on human mood and outlook. Some suggest, for example, that a lack of exposure to sunlight may be linked to feelings of depression in some individuals.

Most of us have probably experienced looking out our window on a blustery, cloudy, winter day and feeling cold and isolated from the rest of the world. The spring's thaw may seem a lifetime away. But you can take a mini-vacation by visiting a local conservatory or zoo. Or better, you can befriend nature in winter by learning to cross-country ski or ice skate, or simply, bundle up and hike a woodsy trail. Learn to co-opt winter if it gets you down. And, remember, the snow melts, the grass and trees return to green, and the sun shines bright and warm again. Allow yourself to be rejuvenated through the power of nature. Open yourself to its healing effects. The cleansing fragrance of an evening rain or the beauty of the rainbow that follows can inspire a quiet peace within you. Discover that part of nature that touches you with its magnificently tranquil power.

If nature is one of your favorite spirit lifters, but it's a drab, gray day, then use your memory to enjoy cheery, yellow daffodils. Through mental imagery, or visualization, you can close your eyes and visit your garden in full bloom, a favorite lakeshore vacation spot, or your neighborhood park.

To enhance this experience, recall with *all* your senses. Remember the earthy *fragrance* of fall leaves, the *sound* of a loon, or water gently lapping onto the lakeshore, and the *feel* of the silky sand at the beach. Through your imagination, the power of nature is always available to you! And to give your imagination a little boost, get a few nature-sounds audio tapes to play as you meditate or fall asleep. Probably dozens of sounds are available: rain, ocean surf, swamp sounds, birds in the forest. Choose whatever appeals to you.

## Art

Art is another rich source of spiritual nourishment. I cannot recommend specific works of art, for the beauty in art is in each individual's interpretation and enjoyment of it. Visit an art gallery or museum. Be open to receiving not only a message from works of art, but also a feeling of inspiration. I will never forget seeing a statue of Joan of Arc in the Cathedral of Notre Dame in Paris. The feeling I got as I looked at that beautiful statue was the feeling of great peace and strength in the face of great adversity and pain. Many years later I met a wonderful woman who reminded me of that work of art and its inspiring message. The woman has painful and crippling arthritis throughout her entire body. But, when one looks into her face, one never sees pain, only peace and gentle strength.

A photograph can inspire. A friend of mine, a cardiologist, recommends exercise to his patients not only for the physical benefit, but also for the spiritual benefit. He believes that one of the most important benefits of exercise is that it increases our self-esteem. In his lectures he uses a slide showing a woman running up a hill. Superimposed on the picture are the words: "The Sound of Cheering from Within." Surely it is her Physician Within who is doing that cheering. I love that picture, and I love my friend for sharing it.

## Altruism

Perhaps the greatest spark we can receive occurs when we are giving of ourselves to others. Dr. Hans Selye called it "altruistic egotism," because he realized that we help ourselves when we help others. Through giving we receive. The spark of your spirit touching my spirit ignites the most powerful force in the universe: Love.

> Someday after mastering the winds, the tides, and gravity,
> We shall harness for God the energy of Love
> and then for the second time in history,
> we shall have discovered Fire.
> —Pierre Teilhard De Chardin

Rabbi Harold Kushner, author of *When Bad Things Happen to Good People*, commented that the most important ingredient in fulfillment is to know that we made a difference. He said it needn't be something great. "Little deeds of loving-kindness make the difference." Rabbi Kushner suggested that just as our bodies are created to require certain kinds of food for good health, "our souls are made so certain kinds of behaviors are healthy for us and other kinds are toxic."

Theologian Paul Tillich gave us insight into the importance of kindness when he said that God is not a benevolent cloud in the sky, separate from all of us "down here." Instead, God is as close as the closest human being is to us. God is in each of us, and we connect with God whenever we communicate a loving message to anyone around us. When we give or receive those loving messages, we experience feelings of warmth and goodness as our Physician Within awakens and stirs. We nourish our spirit whenever, out of love, we:

- say a kind word,
- share a beautiful thought,
- telephone a friend to see how she is,
- bring soup to a neighbor in need,
- spend time with a lonely or hurting person,
- give food, clothing, or money to those in need,
- volunteer our time or talent to a worthy cause,
- hug someone,
- help someone you'll probably never see again, (a stranger in a grocery store, a child thousands of miles away),
- or . . . (continue with your own list).

Perhaps, like me, you will find a lot of overlapping as you think of your Physician Within. See that overlapping as reinforcement. God is surely my invincible summer, my undying song of Hope, and my loving, healing Physician Within.

What is yours? It's there, my friend. Within you lies abundant power to help you make it through any challenge you encounter. Find it. If necessary, get support to help you open up to it. Then, nourish it. Most important, believe in it, because traditional wisdom, human intuition, sacred scriptures, and research findings all reinforce the body, mind, and spirit concept.

## The mystery of the spirit

In opening yourself to the power of the spirit, keep in mind its mystery. This book cannot be a recipe for spiritual healing. It can only begin to help you consider some of its power. However, the greatest power of the spirit is unknown to most of us and cannot be explained. We benefit the most when we let go of our human need to understand and control, when we humbly and honestly recognize our need for a power greater than ourselves.

God meets us in our places of despair—in our questioning hours—as God met Job. After the brokenness, pain, and despair comes healing. That is the mystery of the spirit. It is the power of the spirit that will help you rise above the reality of disease and injury, help you to endure pain, and experience that peace which is beyond human understanding.

The ancient Sanskrit shares this timeless message of well-being:

**Look to this day
for it is the very life of Life.
In its brief course lie all the verities and realities
of your existence.
For yesterday is but a dream
And tomorrow is only a vision
But today well-lived makes
every yesterday a dream of Happiness
and every tomorrow a vision of Hope.
Look well, therefore, to this day.
It is the life of Life!**
—Sanskrit

## Summary

- As unwelcome as they are, pain and disease can teach us self-discovery and result in great spiritual growth.

- 

  Persons without a rich spiritual life may ask life's most profound questions only when faced with a great health challenge. This process often leads to the spiritual domain and may ultimately help one to discover one's Physician Within.

- Your Physician Within can be God, a profound conviction, Faith, Hope, Trust, Peace. Each person defines it differently.

- Philosophy, literature, and religion can help you uncover your source of power and nourish it as well. The only way to activate it, however, is through faith.

- Even with an active internal power, there are still times when we must turn to our external power sources and receive their spark.

- The mystery of the spirit lies in the truth that after the pain and despair comes healing.

## Reflection Questions

1. Define your Physician Within.

2. List the different ways you connect with your Physician Within.

3. Identify the external sparks in your life that you can turn to on the days you feel "down."

# CHAPTER 9

# Make Your Life a Story of Empowerment

Of the many stories I've heard that describe empowered persons, I will begin with two. As you read them please be open to the lesson they have to teach about empowerment, generally, and more important, be aware of the meaning they hold for you in particular.

Ryan White was a young boy who had hemophilia, which required blood transfusions. Through a tainted blood product, Ryan developed AIDS. As if the horror of having this disease was not enough to cope with, he was forbidden by the school board—prompted by public pressure—to attend school. After a long and bitter legal battle, he won the right to attend school, but it shattered his life. He and his mother finally moved to a more tolerant climate. Ryan White is the perfect example of an innocent victim. He could have chosen to become bitter and angry, but instead, he became a champion for the human spirit by traveling around the country, making dozens of public appearances promoting understanding and compassion. The gentle strength with which he lived and died is empowerment.

An example on a smaller scale is the woman with severe and painful arthritis who stood looking hopelessly at her Christmas tree. She wanted to water it, but her stiff knees made it impossible to bend down to pour water into the tree stand. She felt some anger and then determination to solve this problem. She sat down to list all the options that she could think of. The list included calling her neighbor to come over and do it, risking a dry tree until her daughter came to visit in a week. As she lowered her gaze to stare into that space whence ideas cometh, her eyes fell upon the Christmas wrapping paper. That gave her an idea. Carefully she took the remaining paper off the roll. Then, examining the inner core of the Christmas wrap, she discovered just what she had hoped to find—a sturdy funnel through which she could deliver water to her thirsty tree while she remained standing instead of bending or kneeling. The surge of well-being she experienced is an example of empowerment.

## Healthy people are empowered

Years ago, a pediatric endocrinologist asked me, "Who should get diabetes?" He had observed patients who had successfully integrated diabetes and its lifestyle requirements into their lives and went on with life and others who found living with diabetes extremely difficult. So his real question was, "Why do some people do well when confronted with challenges?" And my intuitive response to that question is, "Because they're healthy people."

What does it mean to be a whole and healthy person, and how is that achieved?

Today we use the word *empowerment* to describe the process of discovery that helps us to become a whole and healthy person.

## Defining empowerment

Empowerment is, in our sense, the granting of power or authority to oneself. It is not received from or approved by another. That is essential to understand in this context.

People are empowered when, attempting to solve problems or achieve goals, they access and use their psychological, social, emotional, and spiritual resources. No matter what challenge they face, empowered people exercise control over their own lives. No one, however, is immune to the challenges that threaten our sense of control. Most of us spend our lives getting back into control or working to maintain control over our lives. We do this by continually developing the psychological, social, emotional, and spiritual aspects of our lives. The push that begins this development is often a great life challenge, like the diagnosis of a chronic disease. When people are challenged physically, they seek strength from their other resources. For some, it is a discovery of these resources; for others, a rediscovery; and still others find it an affirmation of what they have valued for some time.

If the challenges in life move us to discover, reconnect with, or affirm our inner resources, then we can see the "blessing in disguise" in an otherwise unwanted life experience. That is why

I like to think of life as "moving ahead through challenge." Because of challenges we move on—developing, discovering, becoming. When people are not challenged, they simply coast through life. This is seen in school when students can get good grades without trying; in work settings when employees continue doing work that does not challenge them. These people could choose to challenge themselves, but it is easier to take the path of least resistance.

However, when people are diagnosed with a chronic health challenge, the choice has been made for them. So where does empowerment fit in when we are clearly not in control of this critical life event? Empowerment emerges when we choose to continue to pursue a fulfilling life in the face of a new and probably frightening physical challenge.

Some people seem to move intuitively and quickly toward empowerment, accessing all their resources and using them to move on with their life. They receive the rewards of empowerment: **strength** to make the journey no matter how steep the climb; **wisdom** to see beyond the momentary challenge of their disease to the growth it can bring; and **hope,** which allows them to respond to their challenge in a positive way—managing their disease while celebrating life.

For many, it is a struggle to incorporate their disease into their life. They may view their disease as a disaster or a burden. It is natural to go through a grieving process similar to that suggested by Elisabeth Kübler-Ross in her work with people grieving the loss of a loved one or preparing to die themselves. The diagnosis of a disease is a loss inasmuch as we grieve the loss of our formerly healthy self. The grieving process includes such stages as denial, anger, fear, sadness, and finally, acceptance. Acceptance is not resignation. Acceptance involves the recognition that, although a disease or health problem may be an unchangeable fact of our life, it is our response to that fact that determines the quality of our lives. I see the stage of acceptance as a sort of "graduation." When we can move beyond the pain and begin to look forward again to life, we have graduated. We are free.

## Understanding empowerment

One of the leading voices on issues relating to empowerment is Bob Anderson, Associate Research Scientist at the University of Michigan Medical School. Pressed to give a one-sentence definition, Bob gave this: "Empowerment is the lived awareness of our human freedom and responsibility." This definition makes the essential point that empowerment can transform the quality of our lives only by *experiencing* it (lived awareness). Merely an intellectual understanding of empowerment is as helpful as a book on food would be to a hungry person.

Learning about love illustrates this point well. People learn the most meaningful lessons about love by loving and being loved— not by reading a book or hearing a lecture about love. Thus, the *process* of becoming empowered is essential to our understanding because it is a lived experience. The process can be described by four words: *explore, reflect, apply, and evaluate.* These four words describe the process even better when they are shown graphically.

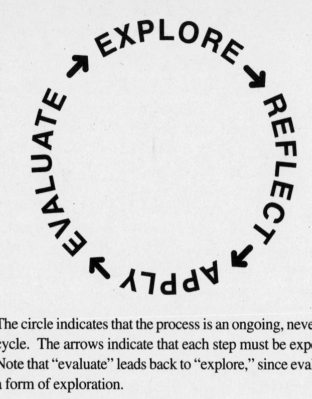

The circle indicates that the process is an ongoing, never-ending cycle. The arrows indicate that each step must be experienced. Note that "evaluate" leads back to "explore," since evaluation is a form of exploration.

*Stories clothe theory in humanity*

Stories are especially useful in helping to describe and understand empowerment because empowerment is about the human dimension of life. I have used stories throughout this book for two reasons: First, they help us to see the connection between theory and humanity, and second, they help each of us to connect with our own humanity. Stories help us to better understand ourselves and others.

**Empowerment springs from the unique experience (story) of the individual, which connects us with the universal experience of being human.**

Our understanding of the world goes from micro to macro. Illustrating this concept is the story of a little boy who was pestering his dad one Sunday to play catch. His dad promised to do so—as soon as he finished reading the newspaper. The little boy kept interrupting his father. Finally, in a desperate attempt to buy some reading time, the father picked up a section of the paper that had a large picture of the globe on it. He tore the picture into many pieces, then gave it to his son, saying, "Go solve the puzzle. Put the picture back together. Then we'll play catch." The boy ran off and his father settled back to read the paper. Shortly, the boy reappeared with the picture of the globe neatly put back together. Astonished at the speed of his son's work, the father asked his boy how he could have done it so quickly. The boy responded by saying, "On the back of the picture of the globe is a picture of a man. It was much easier to put that picture back together than the globe. When the man was right, so was the world."

*Every story has a lesson in it.*

But the particular meaning of a story is created by each person who hears or reads it. Each of us brings our unique personality and history to each life experience (story), and as a result, a meaning emerges that is all our own. As we grow and develop as people, we often find new meaning in old stories. The story of David and Goliath moves from an adventure story to an allegory of good versus evil, to a profoundly meaningful story of what it is to have faith.

A literary hero can chaperone children into adulthood, lending perspective and kindling dreams. Literary heroes can encourage discovery and growth in adults as they explore the world around and within them.

Stories are also to be found in day-to-day life experiences and range from the "yesterday on my way home" variety to the dramatic stories of life and death. Besides teaching us lessons, stories provide us with heroes to inspire and guide us.

The world is full of brave and inspiring people. In January, 1981, when the U.S. hostages from the embassy in Iran were released, a radio commentator said, "Sometimes hanging in there, surviving, is a form of heroism, too." This comment exactly described the kind of heroism those hostages exhibited.

Helen Keller once said, "So much has been given to me that I do not have time to ponder over that which has been denied." Certainly an inspiration to people without hearing or sight, her story is inspiring to us all.

Booker T. Washington said: "I have learned that success is to be measured not so much by the position that one has reached in life, as by the obstacles which one has overcome while trying to succeed." His story taught a nation and the world that obstacles uncover the greatness of the human spirit. It is the stories of real people that give life to such instructive thoughts as this, by John W. Gardner:

We are not at our best perched at the summit; we are climbers, at our best, when the way is steep.

The story of *when* Thanksgiving became a national holiday encourages reflection on what it means to be thankful. In the midst of the Civil War, one of the greatest tragedies of our country, Abraham Lincoln paused to permanently dedicate one day a year to giving thanks for our national and personal blessings.

Stories are gifts, which only a loss of memory can destroy. They provide a means to the end Ralph Waldo Emerson spoke of:

> Though we travel the world over to find the beautiful, we must carry it with us or we find it not." Our stories become part of us and can be called upon at a moment's notice to entertain, guide, or inspire. I read about an 80-year-old woman who is blind. She made this insightful comment: "People should furnish their minds well. If I have to sit alone, at least I can sit in my own well-furnished mind.

Joseph Campbell described the universal aspect of our shared humanity through his study of the stories of heroes. From the Bible, from Greek mythology, from virtually every known culture, Campbell studied what he called the hero's journey. And he said we are all heroes, following our own journeys. I like the journey metaphor for empowerment, because it reinforces the idea that empowerment is an ongoing process. The path has peaks and valleys, flowers and poison ivy. We cope with some things and celebrate others. But we keep moving forward. And journey suggests the words "quest" and "question," both derived from the same Latin word for "seek." This seems appropriate, since questions usually start and continue our journeys.

*Ask questions about your life.*

Follow where the questions lead you. It is the questions that lead us on our journey. The crises of life evoke the big questions, which can then take us to the most interesting places. One such crisis is middle age, when people begin to wonder whether what they have experienced in life is enough. "What is my life all about?" one may ask. Another such crisis can be the diagnosis of a chronic disease with its attendant questions of "Why me?" and "What will this mean to my ongoing enjoyment of life?"

The initial questions that arise may be like a knee-jerk reaction. They often tend to be either superficial or the sort of questions one has read about or heard others express. They are almost an expression of shock. But the later questions, those reflecting deeper thinking, are more likely to become our teachers. Among the most profound are: "What is this trying to teach me? How can I use this experience for growth?"

Joseph Campbell referred to crisis as the "call to adventure." A crisis can begin an adventure of learning and growth.

*Listen for the lessons.*

To listen for lessons is to have faith that there are lessons to be learned. Such an openness allows for finding lessons in the unlikeliest places and receiving gifts you would never have suspected were even there.

After the first edition of *The Physician Within* was published, I appeared on several talk shows to introduce it. On one nationally syndicated television show, there were three of us as guests. In the middle of the interview, the hostess suddenly turned to the camera and announced: "Now we're going to take a four-minute commercial break. During the break I will randomly select three people from the audience and assign them to our three guests. Then, I'll send them all backstage, where our experts will solve their problems and come back and tell us about it." There was no time to protest. But I did manage to fend off the sheer panic that would have been so natural to feel. I realized that I had to keep my wits about me. I clearly did not see this situation as a call to adventure, that is, an opportunity to learn and grow. My only thought was survival.

I stood backstage with the woman who had been assigned to me. I said, "Tell me about you." She immediately frowned and said, "I have terminal cancer. My doctor put me on one medication which made me violently sick. Then he put me on another, which was even worse." We were now at 3 minutes and 15 seconds out of the allotted four minutes. I said, "Forgive me for interrupting, but our time is short. Instead of telling me what hasn't worked, tell me what has. You look wonderful. How are you making it?"

The minute I asked that question, the frown disappeared, her shoulders went back and she said, "That doctor told me I had 6 months to live... and that was 18 months ago. I told him, 'Young man, my husband and I go to Florida every winter and we're going this winter.' In fact, we've been back twice since the 'death sentence.' That first winter back, each morning before I even opened my eyes, I would visualize myself walking on the beach. I felt the cool, wet sand under my feet, felt the breeze in my face, smelled the salty air, and heard the sea gulls. Then, I'd open my eyes and go do that."

In this unlikely place and situation, I *had* received a call to adventure. I learned a new appreciation for an old lesson: Our time is indeed short, whether it is four minutes "backstage" or 94 years on the planet. And we have choices about how we will live our time. That determined woman did not give up when she was told she had cancer. She chose to be in control of her life. She personifies for me the memorable quote by Aldous Huxley: "Experience is not what happens to you; it's what you do with what happens to you."

And sometimes there are gifts for us hidden away in our questions.

I never have understood the answer to the question of why I lost my father when I was a child. But as an adult, I came to learn how to draw strength from that loss. I mentioned earlier about the hazard of too much rainfall for crops, citing that plants that have easy access to water do not have to send their roots deep to find water. I remember hearing that the first time, realizing that without a deep root, plants are easily uprooted by the winds and storms. I remember that as soon as I heard that explanation, the proverbial light bulb went on. "That's why I'm strong as an adult," I thought. "Because when I was just a little sprout, my roots had to go very deep in order to find the river of life."

It is those "Aha!" experiences that provide life-transforming empowerment. That's why it is our own personal stories that are the basis of our empowerment. One of the values in hearing other people's stories lies in their ability to connect us to our own.

Sometimes literature can connect us to our own stories. A poem—the title of which I've never known—by Rainer Maria

Rilke has had profound meaning for me. In it, he counsels us to be patient with all the unresolved questions in our lives and learn to not only *live* those questions but to actually *love* them. He suggests if you do that you will "live along someday into the answers."

The reason this poem means so much to me is that it makes me think of my own story, which ranges over many years. When I was a teenager, I developed a discoloration on my leg. I found out that it was *necrobiosis lipoidica diabeticorum*. My doctor was quick to point out how lucky I was. It was my only complication of diabetes, and it wasn't serious. It was "only ugly." To a teenaged girl, there's no such thing as "only ugly." I hated having "NLD," but I adapted to it by owning about ten dozen pairs of knee socks. Over time it faded and as I matured, it became less of an issue, until after our son, John, was born and seriously injured by the erroneous IV solution. After two major plastic surgeries before he turned four years old, John had hideous scars on his leg—purple, jagged, bumpy scars.

The summer he was three-and-a-half, John and I were sitting outside with our bare legs stretched out in front of us. He noticed the very faint residual discoloration on my leg and said, "Mommy, what's that?" I replied by saying, "Oh, Mommy has a funny spot on her leg." Then, with a look on his face somewhere between serene and matter-of-fact, he turned his gaze to his own leg, shrugged his little shoulders and said, "Johnny has a funny spot on his leg too." And, at that moment, all I could think was, "Thank you, God, for necrobiosis lipoidica diabeticorum."

## The pillars of empowerment

*Awareness* and *choice* are two of the four pillars of empowerment. We need to be aware of who we are as human beings. This awareness includes insight into our values, goals, needs, and problems. It includes awareness of our personal history, of the various cultures that have influenced us and our health beliefs. Awareness makes it possible for us to make informed choices.

The diagnosis of a chronic disease can bring to the surface an awareness of what we *value*. Many of the questions that initially occur to people center around what their disease will mean in their pursuit of a fulfilling life. In addition to their values, people become more aware of their *goals* as their disease presents a threat to their health and well-being. The integration of a disease into one's life occurs over time as people discover ways to pursue what they value, continue to set goals, and solve their problems.

During the lengthy and involved process of integrating the disease into a life they perceive as worth living, people discover their *needs*. They discover the *need to adapt, to solve problems, to stay motivated, to bolster their self-image, to manage stress, to find support, and to maintain hope.* This discovery leads them into the lifelong exploration designed to continue meeting those needs. The best education programs offered are those that promote this exploration, but no class in the world can do it quite like life experience. In daily life, we find the resources that fill our needs, thus facilitating the process linking person, disease, and life.

The other two pillars of empowerment are *freedom* and *responsibility*. That we are both free and responsible is a basic idea of the empowerment philosophy. *We are free to make our choices and yet responsible for the consequences of those choices.* We are free to choose to act or react. If this statement seems a bit daunting, please keep in mind that you empower yourself by using all of your resources. Review your resources whenever you begin to feel overwhelmed. Facing the challenge is not something you must do alone. In addition to your own inner resources, you can call on outside resources like family, friends, health professionals, clergy, counselors, teachers. The *empowered* person *accesses* and *uses* available resources and works at developing additional resources.

## Tell your stories

One way to discover your resources is to tell a story using the subject of each chapter in this book as a theme. Then add themes of your own.

The story can be an actual event from your life, or it can be pure fiction. Either way, it is likely to be instructive for you—helping you to better understand yourself and the resources you have to help you meet your challenge.

A nurse in the pediatric burn unit of a hospital described how storytelling helped her young patients. Originally intended as a way to distract them from their pain, the stories actually helped the children to tap into their strength and courage.

One little girl chose to visit the jungle as the setting for her story. Once there, she saw a giraffe whose spots were purple (similar to the burns on her legs). The girl said the purple spots made the giraffe easier to find when her friends wanted to play. And during each subsequent appointment, the story was continued from where it had been left before. The giraffe demonstrated courage in saving her friends from hunters. There were stories depicting love and concern, strength and determination, and hope.

Whether a story begins with the personal pronoun "I" or a fictionalized character like the giraffe, you are the hero of the story. Tell your stories to friends or relatives (and share theirs) or simply write them in a journal. This process of storytelling will help you to discover both your resources and your weaknesses. Once you have gathered this information, you can decide whether a problem needs to be solved or a goal needs to be set.

**Threats to empowerment**

As you explore and reflect on the resources that can help you further develop into a healthy, empowered person, also explore and reflect on the forces that threaten your empowerment. Some of the common threatening forces are fear, anger, ignorance, hopelessness, and misguided help.

Each of the above forces can rob people of empowerment by becoming the power that controls their life. As you read through the following, reflect on your stories. Become aware of the areas in your life (the chapters in your story) that are influenced by forces that threaten your ability to be in control of your own life.

Then reflect on the resources around and within you that can help you to take and keep control.

*Fear*

It is natural to experience fear at points throughout life. It can be healthy if it warns us of an impending danger and helps us to make a responsible decision to avoid the danger. But fear can be crippling if it takes control of life.

When people are diagnosed with a chronic disease, it is natural to experience fear. Many diseases pose a real threat to one's life and well-being. The Health Belief Model states that people must be aware of the seriousness of their disease and their personal vulnerability in order to take responsible action. That's the positive aspect of fear. Fear becomes negative when it immobilizes. So, on a day-to-day basis, we can choose to focus on life and a commitment to living each day fully, instead of on the "what ifs" and potential problems.

If you sense that fear is a problem for you right now, explore it. What are you fearful of? Disease-related questions need to be explored with a knowledgeable and caring health professional. Fears related to more personal issues can be explored with the help of a friend who is a good listener or by interacting with people who have the same disease. Local chapters of health agencies like Heart, Diabetes, Cancer, Lupus, and Arthritis provide opportunities for just such interaction.

I have been a volunteer with the American Diabetes Association for many years. My involvement has provided me with many opportunities to meet wonderful people. I have been particularly inspired by a woman with whom I have done committee work and who I now am privileged to call a dear friend. Like me, Kathy Plumb has diabetes. But our experience with diabetes has been different. I am relatively free of its complications. Kathy has experienced blindness, kidney failure, a heart attack, hearing impairment, and significant nerve damage.

My fears about diabetes have centered on complications like these and what they would mean to the quality of my life. Getting to know Kathy as a person has been extraordinarily helpful to me. Through a conscious decision, she has taken the circumstances of her life—incredible physical challenges—and integrated them with her *values* of serving others, her *need* to find meaning and fulfillment, and her *personal history*, which includes a strong faith, a close-knit family, and good friends. Kathy contributes to the community by serving on various boards and committees. She is admired and respected for her professional work, which is motivational speaking. She enjoys her marriage and a long list of friends and activities. Because she has successfully integrated challenges and a fulfilling life, she is one of my shining examples of empowerment. Her example has helped me to let go of fear and regain my faith that I, too, could continue to pursue what is important to me if I were to experience complications of diabetes.

A man whose sister had died from the complications of diabetes was unable to overcome fear when he was diagnosed with diabetes. He was convinced that what happened to his sister would happen to him. He didn't share his fear with his medical team. Their view of him was that he was an otherwise healthy person who could manage his disease with all of the latest technology and education. He took classes and bought the blood monitoring device and never used either the information or the tools. He was so fearful he would die soon anyway that he did nothing to prevent that from happening. And his daily life was lived in desperation as he ate extravagantly, drank heavily, and smoked cigarettes with the full knowledge that he was courting disaster. *Fear* became the power in control of his life.

## Anger

Another threat to empowerment is anger. Anger robs us of empowerment if we get stuck in it and fail to move forward with our lives. Psychologist John E. Valusek, Ph.D., founder of People are Not for Hitting—an organization to reduce misguided anger and violent behavior—told a story about a patient newly diagnosed with cancer whom he was asked to visit. He found a woman withdrawn and bitter. As he talked with her, she told him that her bitterness was caused by cancer. He asked her how much time she had to live.

Startled by the question, she admitted she didn't know. He asked her if she expected to be alive for his visit the next day. Impatiently, she responded that she would be. He kept asking her to say how long she expected to live, boosting his questions by a week and then a month. Finally, she told him that she fully expected to live for a year. Then he asked her if she intended to live each of the remaining 364 days with the anger and bitterness of today. His question brought her an awareness of what she was doing and what choices she really had. Although she didn't change her attitude overnight, she began the change that eventually led her to explore and discover new choices. Even though she had cancer, she still had to decide how she would live each of her remaining days.

Anger can be the springboard to empowerment if we turn its energy into determination to solve problems. A young mother was concerned for her six-month-old baby. He slept fitfully on her shoulder and cried incessantly when she laid him in his crib. When he refused to nurse at the breast, she became worried and took him to the doctor. She was sent home with the admonition, "If you had five chilren, you wouldn't worry so much."

Two days later, she returned to the doctor because the baby was no better. This time the doctor suggested that she needed to see a psychiatrist. Her worry for her baby turned to anger. She went home and called a university hospital in a nearby city. She announced that she was bringing in a very sick baby, and they should be prepared to receive him. Upon her arrival, it was determined that, in fact, her baby was critically ill. He underwent emergency surgery and was saved. Anger can be empowering. Or it can be crippling. How we make use of it is our choice.

Fear and anger can return uninvited throughout our lifetime. As the circumstances of life change, our health challenge gets woven in and must be dealt with—sometimes creating turmoil. When life insurance was denied to me because I have diabetes, I responded with anger. I was angry at a system that would not look at individuals.

The doctor who had examined me for the insurance company had congratulated me on being so healthy, yet insurance was denied just because of the diagnosis of diabetes. I was angry because my husband and I had the same needs (and, I felt, rights) as any young couple. I was at home with our baby, and if I were killed in an accident, the cost of child care would be out of reach for my husband, who made a modest teacher's salary.

Along with the anger, I felt fear. It's like living in a house not covered by fire insurance. The "what ifs" are terrible. Empowerment returns when you take action—like checking the wiring on a house and following general, sound, safety measures. I practiced healthful living. I experienced again the need to approach life with practicality and faith. I also took action by working with the American Diabetes Association for sensible reform in the insurance industry. Through responsible action, I experienced a change in attitude from anger to determination and hope.

As of this writing, the insurance situation has not changed entirely. But, even if the problem does not get solved, we can resolve uncomfortable feelings of anger or fear. We become empowered when we commit to working on the solving of a problem, by assuming responsibility for our own life.

## Ignorance

Ignorance is like a shadow, and *knowledge* is the light that banishes it. The most empowered person imaginable probably won't manage a chronic disease very well unless part of that person's storehouse of resources is knowledge about the disease and about its management. But history has shown us that knowledge of the disease alone has not been enough to help people change their lifestyle behaviors to manage their disease. Nor has knowledge about disease been known to promote health and well-being. Empowerment education emphasizes the life skills that people need to be healthy people. Combined with knowledge about managing the disease, empowerment education helps people to balance the requirements of their disease with their own "requirements" for a fulfilling life.

Knowledge leads to awareness. It is impossible to take responsibility for influences in our life if we are not aware of them. **Empowered people make informed choices—informed by an awareness of all the forces coming into play in the choices they face**. To be empowered to live well with a chronic disease requires knowledge about disease-related issues, as well as the skills and attributes of human health and well-being.

*Hopelessness*

Our vulnerability to hopelessness continues for a lifetime. That's why we need to have an understanding of the source of our hope, how to access it, and how to nourish it. Refer to the "Physician Within" chapter for a review of this process.

Hope is at the very heart of our humanity. It can be both inspiring and affirming to learn about the struggles and triumphs of others who are able to move from hopelessness to hope. Because hope is part of all humanity, we can find stories anywhere in the world. Vaclav Havel was imprisoned in Czechoslovakia, the country of which he later became president. His comment on hope:

> Hope is a state of mind, not of the world...Hope, in this deep and powerful sense, is not the same as joy that things are going well, or willingness to invest in enterprises that are

obviously heading for success, but rather an ability to work for something because it is good, not just because it stands a chance to succeed.

I was inspired by Havel's words when I found myself in a difficult situation. I had served for ten years on the Board of Governors of an inner-city hospital in Minneapolis. Because of the economic difficulties in health care, our hospital was having to close. There was a collective community grieving as we prepared for its closing. I remember our final board meeting. I looked around the table at men and women from business, medicine, religion, education, and government. They were not only leaders of the community but also people who had given of themselves to this wonderful hospital, which just eight weeks earlier had received the highest commendation from its accrediting organization, the Joint Commission of the Accreditation of Hospitals.

We could not understand. In attempting to understand, we spoke of the "integrity of the spirit" that results from working on something because it is so worthy of our efforts—even if "success" is not to be the outcome. It was during that conversation that the following story found its way into the board room and into our hearts:

It seems that a United States senator interviewed Mother Teresa. He said to her, "Mother Teresa, I'm sorry to say this to you, but it's hopeless. What you are doing is hopeless. No matter how hard you work, millions of people will die." Mother Teresa's remarkable response was: "God does not require that I be successful. He asks that I be faithful."

*Misguided help*

Sometimes the very people who love us the most and who want to help end up hindering our progress instead. Parents of children with chronic disease are a classic example. Unable to trade places with their child, they mistakenly do what they think is the next best thing: completely take over their child's self-care. In their mind, it is the best thing they can do, but it may make the child dependent instead of preparing the child for independence.

There is a fine line between the appropriate support that fosters responsible self-care in the child and the smothering support that removes the child from responsibility, creating an unhealthy reliance on others instead of self. On either side of appropriate support are two potentially dangerous extremes. One is when the parents do too much; the other extreme is when they adopt a laissez-faire attitude, saying, in essence, "This is your disease. If it's going to get managed, you'll have to do it."

I remember talking with the mother of a seven-year-old girl with diabetes. The mother was frustrated that her daughter wasn't ready to assume full responsibility for her diabetes. Seven is mighty young for such responsibility.

The pediatric health professionals with whom I have worked help parents through a staged approach of offering their child support. The most intense parental involvement occurs at the diagnosis of the disease and when children are very young. In the staged approach to support, parents gradually back off as they give the child increasing responsibility. The parents decide when to cut back on their activity after consulting the child's medical team and having a dialogue with their child. Respect for the child's readiness is an essential part of the child's empowerment. It teaches the balance of independence and interdependence. Interdependence is the normal and healthy need to both give and receive support.

The issues are quite similar for adults, except that parental involvement is replaced by family, such as spouse and children. Adults can be robbed of empowerment by an overly protective spouse or overly solicitous children. And adults are just as vulnerable to loneliness as children are if they feel a lack of support. The term "codependency" has been used to describe the situation in which people have an unhealthy need to depend on others who have an equally unhealthy need to have others depend on them.

Health professionals are equally liable to rob rather than encourage empowerment. The irony is that they intend to help. Because of their training and the culture they are part of, health professionals want to fix problems. Their professional reward comes from "making it better." Their compassionate natures are reinforced when they see the problem resolved. However, if people are to be truly empowered, they must solve their own problems. In the days when most of the health problems that were presented to doctors were infectious diseases or broken bones, it was entirely appropriate for the health professional to fix the problems. But today, most of the health problems that doctors see are chronic in nature. They cannot be fixed. It is up to the people who have the disease to solve problems relating to their disease on a daily and sometimes an hourly basis. It is not only impractical to expect health professionals to solve daily problems, it is impossible. The supportive health professional role was discussed in the "Support" chapter. Here, as we reflect on empowerment and the health professional's role, explore how well you feel your medical team does in encouraging your empowerment. The following football metaphor describes a situation in which a quarterback was knowledgeable but not empowered to make use of that knowledge.

A coach decided to send a totally inexperienced quarterback into a football game they were losing. He cavalierly advised the young quarterback to call play #44 twice and then to punt. The team was on their own 4 yard line. The quarterback did as he was told. He called play #44, and it worked! The team advanced 45 yards down field. He called the play again and it worked again, advancing the team to within five yards of their opponent's end zone. The quarterback then called for a punt as he had been told.

When the young quarterback came off the field, the coach grabbed him by the shoulder pads and demanded, "What was going through your mind?!" The quarterback shrugged and said, "All I could think of was what a dumb coach I have."

For years we have used the term "therapeutic alliance" to describe an effective relationship between a patient and the health care team. It requires communication between the two to develop a working partnership with just the right balance. Some patients feel comfortable making medication adjustments because their health care provider has taught them how to do it appropriately. Other patients do not feel comfortable making such decisions.

Each "alliance" needs to consider the people involved and meet everyone's needs.

## Compliance versus the empowerment model

The empowerment model in health care and patient education is offered as an alternative to a compliance-based medical model. For many years patients were simply told what to do (take this medication; follow this diet) and were expected to comply (do exactly as they were told). The compliance model does not take into account the fact that people make their own choices. But we do. And our choices are based upon our values, goals, needs, and problems as *human beings*.

Successful management of a disease must take into account the human dimension. Without the human dimension, people with chronic diseases become diabetics, athritics, or epileptics, instead of *people* who have diabetes, arthritis, or epilepsy. In the empowerment model, people are encouraged to focus on life. They are aware of their disease and its requirements, but they are devoted to the pursuit of a fulfilling life. This does *not* mean they ignore their disease. It means they are *aware* of both their life goals and the goals related to managing their disease. They integrate the needs of their disease into the pursuit of a fulfilling life. They've accepted the fact that their disease is part of their life, and they adapt their life to accommodate it.

In the compliance model, the power was thought to rest solely with the health professionals. However, the fragile quality of such power became evident as soon as the patient said, "I'm not going to do that." Sometimes actions speak even louder than words, and a subsequent appointment shows that "orders" have not been followed. Frustration for everyone involved was often the result.

What has emerged is an empowerment model that divides the power and responsibility between patient and health professional. This model acknowledges that patients cannot be forced to follow a lifestyle dictated by health-care professionals. This change is reflected in the language we use to describe the behavior of patients—now commonly referred to as "clients." While in the past it was common to speak of noncompliance and behavior modification, the empowerment model speaks of self-awareness, personal responsibility, informed choices, and quality of life.

The power is split between health professional and client according to the "specialty" of each. The health professional is seen as the medical expert who shares knowledge of and expertise about a specific disease. The client is seen as the expert on his or her own life. Today we hear the term "team approach" applied to healing and well-being. The client is no longer a passive member of the team who simply takes orders. The client is a primary decision-maker who makes choices and decisions and then has some of the primary responsibility in carrying out those decisions.

The compliance model is problem-focused. Health insurance promotes the focus on problems because most of them require the diagnosis of a problem in order to cover a clinic or hospital visit. Empowerment is concerned with preventing problems. In the compliance model, a visit to a mental health professional could not be made unless or until there was a diagnosable problem. In the empowerment model, people with chronic diseases would be given the opportunity to explore healthy coping strategies so that problems could be prevented.

There is a pervasive disease orientation in the compliance model, whereas the empowerment model is oriented toward human issues. I once heard a psychologist speak to a group of people with diabetes. The lecture was on stress management, which is vitally important because stress can worsen diabetes, and negative coping methods like eating, drinking, and smoking further compromise health. But, instead of the lecture being on coping methods or anything else of a practical nature, it focused on the hormones involved in the stress response—where they come from and what they do. As I listened I thought: "How is this going to help the next time someone has a fight with a spouse or a boss?" In the classic compliance model, it is physical issues that receive attention. In the empowerment approach, it is the psychological, social, and spiritual.

In an *empowerment approach*, whole person health would be automatically assessed in every person diagnosed with a chronic disease. If the assessment showed needs in coping strategies, support system, or personal capacity for hope, then an intervention would be offered such as peer counseling (talking with someone who lives well with the same challenge), professional counseling, or empowerment education.

For an empowerment model to be most effective, it would be incorporated directly into disease education—helping people to integrate their disease and its management into a healthy, fulfilling life. Additionally, it would be helpful for people who have a specific disease to be visited by a person who has the same disease and who represents the health agency dedicated to that disease (e.g., American Diabetes, Heart, Arthritis, Lupus, MS, Cancer, Lung, etc.). This approach would introduce people to another person who experiences the same challenge, and it would make people aware of the community resources available.

We're a long way from understanding all that we need to about empowerment. It is human nature to look for simple answers or cookbook approaches to fixing problems. But empowerment is a **process** that lasts a lifetime, an **outcome** to be attained time and time again. To those seeking an answer to the question, "Why are people not empowered?" I offer this "simple" response: It is because of a lack of support, a negative set of subcultures, a poor self-image, negative coping mechanisms, feelings of powerlessness, bad habits, hopelessness, and the very chronicity of their disease, which leads to falling off the wagon from time to time.

Chronic diseases last a long time. Throughout their course they can create additional problems. Concurrently, life presents new challenges. The person with a chronic disease is faced with the ongoing challenges of both disease and life.

Empowerment is a **process** that helps people make their journey by facilitating self-awareness, learning, and growth. And when people make choices freely and responsibly, the **outcome** is empowerment.

The process of empowering ourselves never ends. We always have new goals, new problems, new solutions. These goals, problems, and solutions lead to new growth. When growth wanes or stops, we need to start the process again. You can start that process by reviewing each chapter of this book and responding to the questions at the end of each chapter. Or you can get the process going again by using the Plan of Action in the final chapter.

To make empowerment a natural part of your life, try keeping its four major concepts in mind and applying them in your daily life. Again, they are:

**Awareness, choice, freedom, responsibility**

**Awareness** of our values, goals, needs, and problems leads us to make our **choices.** We are **free** to make our own choices, and we are **responsible** for the consequences of our choices.

Choosing our response to life determines the quality of our life. To encourage your reflection and self-application, I close with, of course, a story.

> In the grocery store one day, I approached the check-out line. The woman at the cash register is someone I see regularly. She seemed happy to see me and greeted me warmly. Then she leaned toward me and said softly, "Boy, are the people here today crabby. I don't know what their problem is, but I don't choose to be crabby." We had a brief but pleasant encounter, then I left.
>
> As I walked toward my car, I thought about the choices we each make in how we will experience life. I thought about a friend of mine who has post-polio syndrome. She experiences pain surrounded by uncertainty. No one knows what to expect from post-polio syndrome. Sharon has pain today and no idea what tomorrow will bring.

The last time I saw Sharon we chatted. As we parted, she called out to me, "Make it a good day." It is a choice.

## Summary

- Empowerment is the granting of power or authority to oneself. People become empowered when they use all their resources—psychological, social, emotional, and spiritual—to solve their own problems or achieve their own goals.

- How well we move beyond pain and disease, through the grieving process, to acceptance determines the quality of our lives.

- It is healthy to ask questions about your life and wise to listen carefully for the lessons.

- The four pillars of empowerment are awareness, choice, freedom, and responsibility. In order to make informed choices, we must be aware of ourselves as human beings, of our values and needs and of the forces that influence us. We are free to choose and yet responsible for the consequences of those choices.

- Explore the forces that threaten your empowerment—fear, anger, ignorance, hopelessness, and misguided help.

- As patients, we need to get out of the compliance model, in which all power rests with the physician and other health professionals, and get into the empowerment model, in which power is divided between ourselves and the health professionals.

- The process of empowering ourselves never ends; it is an ongoing lifetime effort.

## Reflection Questions

1. Define empowerment.

2. Place yourself in these situations. Reflect on how you would feel and what you would do.

   **A.** You have arthritis. Some friends invite you to a concert. You are not sure if the concert hall has a ramp, which you require because you cannot climb steps. You don't know whether or not to accept their invitation.

   How would an empowered person respond?

   How would an unempowered person respond?

   **B.** You are visiting with your health care team. They suggest a new health management program for you. Although you see the benefits of this program, you have some concerns about the amount of time and energy it will take to adjust to it.

   How would an empowered person respond?

   How would an unempowered person respond?

3. The key concepts in empowerment are: awareness, choice, freedom and responsibility. Discuss how each of these concepts can be applied to the two situations described in question number 2.

4. Identify which specific forces threaten your sense of control. (See pages 216 to 227.)

5. Discuss which internal or external resources you can use to overcome these threats the next time you experience them.

# Your Plan for Action!

T he end of this book signals the beginning of your journey. See your progress toward wellness along the minus 100 to plus 100 continuum. Decide what you are progressing toward. Although we may all agree that it is a generic "fulfilling life," you will want to use a word or words that are particularly meaningful for you. Is that plus 100 empowerment? Well-being? A good life? Success? Peace? You decide.

Then hold that goal in your heart as you experience daily life. Your experiences may include any of the many mud slides of life, which bring you to the left, and possibly back to zero or worse. The hope for and belief in your goal will help you to get back on track. You can move again toward your goal using the skills presented in this book:

Choosing a wellness approach to all of life's challenges
Building a positive self-image
Motivating yourself to maintain healthy behaviors
    and a hopeful outlook
Adapting to life's constant change
Managing stress positively; working at prevention
Finding solutions to your problems
Activating your support system
Knowing that your Physician Within will keep you going
Making your life a story of empowerment

To encourage action, each chapter ends with questions with a behavioral focus. Knowing the problem-solving process will not help you unless you use it. Take action. Review the summaries and questions at the end of each chapter whenever you sense you are sliding toward the minus 100. To take a preventive approach, I suggest you review the summaries and questions quarterly. Write a note on your calendar to do this review every three months.

Another suggestion is to use the Plan of Action outlined at the end of this chapter. Use it as a comprehensive goal-setting exercise. It begins with your overall goal—stated in the words that give the concept of a fulfilling life your own personal meaning.

The next step is to list the objectives that will lead toward the achievement of your goal. List these objectives as behaviors and be as specific as possible. For example,

I will read nourishing thoughts ten minutes each day.
I will write in my journal five minutes each day.

Some people find it helpful to list general healthy lifestyle behaviors. These can include but are not limited to: wearing seat belts, daily rest and relaxation, taking regular vacations, being smoke-free and drug free, managing stress positively, engaging in regular physical activity, and of course, eating nutritiously. The last three are not only general recommendations, they may be mandated because of your health challenge. If that is the case, keep both a problem prevention *and* health promotion perspective. It will increase your motivation to eat a low-fat meal plan if you recognize that it can help to prevent more heart problems. But, if your focus remains on the problem, you can run the risk of feeling like a martyr or a victim. A health promotion perspective helps you view what you are doing as healthy and wise and, thus, encourages you to feel that way.

Your personal Plan of Action may include some additional behaviors to meet your special needs. These may be specific exercises, physical therapy, a particular meal plan, medications, or various other treatment to enhance your well-being. Because I have diabetes, my additional healthy behaviors include taking insulin and monitoring my own blood sugars.

With even the best laid plan, there are obstacles to be encountered. It can help to reflect ahead of time on what you think those obstacles may be. Some may be related to your challenge or its treatment. Pain may make your prescribed exercise difficult. The effects of chemotherapy may make positive thinking seem like an impossibility. Obstacles related to your humanness include unresolved anger ("I'm not going to take care of this disease. I don't want it!"), lack of motivation ("I know I 'should' do this, but . . ."), discouragement ("I can't keep going. It's more than I can take."), and many, many others. Be realistic in identifying your obstacles.

Revisit the process described in the Problem Solving chapter.

Finding support will also help you overcome obstacles. Your Plan of Action needs lots of support so you have the necessary encouragement and motivation. List your external supports—your sources of help and encouragement, and describe your internal support—your Physician Within.

Include a reward system in your plan. Promise yourself a reward for following the healthy behaviors you have set for yourself.

Finally, know your distress signs. What signs tell you that you are headed down the wrong path? Missing your doctor appointments? Skipping exercise sessions? Forgetting to take your medication? Dwelling on negative thoughts? Feeling sorry for yourself? These are all one-way signs pointing to the minus 100 on the wellness continuum. After identifying your signs of distress, determine where you will go to get the support or the boost you need to get yourself going again in the right direction. The following pages contain several blank Plans of Action. Fill one in for yourself right now. Then use the others whenever you feel a need to get your life back in balance, focused on well-being. I have filled in the first one as an example.

Your Plan of Action is your personalized road map. Enjoy your journey, for the joy is in the quest—the growth—the ongoing discovery and not the destination. We are travelers, you and I. Our destinations may be different. Our detours will be different.

But our purpose is the same: to live well. It is not disease that brings us together. It is our desire and hope for well-being.

I close with another "spark," and I wish you well.

> We are all travelers.
> From birth to death,
> we travel between the eternities.
> May these days be
> pleasant for you, profitable for society,
> Helpful to those you meet, and a joy
> to those who know and love you best.

# Plan of Action

My goal is to live well. To me this means:

*To feel well and have enough physical, mental, emotional,
and spiritual energy to engage fully in life.*

In order to reach my goal, I will follow these healthy lifestyle
behaviors: regular exercise, nutritious eating habits, effective
stress management, and:

*the cultivation of friendships and spiritual development.*

Because I have special needs I will also follow these healthy
behaviors:

*blood glucose monitoring, taking insulin, seeing my MD
regularly.*

Obstacles I may encounter include:

*erratic timing for meals, rich food, and getting too busy to
exercise or meditate.*

I will overcome these obstacles by:

*planning ahead, anticipating.*


My resources for support include:

*family, friends, and faith.*


My rewards for following a healthy lifestyle include:

*short term: buying a new outfit.*
*long term: feeling well, the achievement of my goal.*


My distress signs are:

*using negative coping techniques, high blood glucose results.*


When I notice a distress sign, I will:

*go to my support resources and get back into positive coping techniques.*

# Plan of Action

My goal is to live well. To me this means:

In order to reach my goal, I will follow these healthy lifestyle behaviors: regular exercise, nutritious eating habits, effective stress management, and:

Because I have special needs I will also follow these healthy behaviors:

Obstacles I may encounter include:

I will overcome these obstacles by:

My resources for support include:

My rewards for following a healthy lifestyle include:

My distress signs are:

When I notice a distress sign, I will:

# INDEX